OVERCOMING
THYROID
DISORDERS

second edition

David Brownstein, M.D.

For further copies of <u>Overcoming Thyroid Disorders 2nd Edition</u>:

Call **(888) 647-5616** or send a check or money order for $20.00

($15.00 + $5.00 S+H) or for Michigan residents $20.90 ($15.00 +

$5.00 S&H + $.90 sales tax) to:

> Medical Alternatives Press
> 4173 Fieldbrook Rd.
> West Bloomfield, MI 48323

Or, visit our website at: **www.drbrownstein.com**

Medical Alternatives Press
4173 Fieldbrook Rd.
West Bloomfield, MI 48323
(888) 647-5616
www.drbrownstein.com

Acknowledgements

I would like to thank my editors for helping me put this book together. My wife Allison and Jan Darnell have tirelessly read and re-read it and corrected my English. I cannot thank you enough.

I also wish to thank my sister, Linda Laird, Robert Radtke, Angela Doljevic, Stephanie Buist, and my partners Jeff Nusbaum and Rick Ng for reading and sharing their comments with me.

I can't forget my daughters, Hailey and Jessica for helping me put it together. Thank you girls!!!

Finally, thank you to Ashley Caza and her creative ideas and hard work on the cover design.

About The Author

David Brownstein, M.D. is a Board-Certified family physician who utilizes the best of conventional and alternative therapies. He is the Medical Director for the Center for Holistic Medicine in West Bloomfield, MI. He is a graduate of the University of Michigan and Wayne State University School of Medicine. Dr. Brownstein is a member of the American Academy of Family Physicians and the American College for the Advancement in Medicine. He is the father of two beautiful girls, Hailey and Jessica, and is a retired soccer coach. Dr. Brownstein has lectured internationally about his success using natural items. Dr. Brownstein has authored eight books: *Iodine: Why You Need It, Why You Can't Live Without It, 3rd Edition; Drugs That Don't Work and Natural Therapies That Do; The Miracle of Natural Hormones 3rd Edition; Overcoming Thyroid Disorders 2nd Edition; Overcoming Arthritis; Salt Your Way to Health; The Guide To Healthy Eating;* and *The Guide to a Gluten-Free Diet.*

Dr. Brownstein's office is located at:

Center for Holistic Medicine
5821 W. Maple Rd.
Ste. 192
West Bloomfield, MI 48322
248.851.1600
www.drbrownstein.com
www.centerforholisticmedicine.com

A Word of Caution to the Reader

The information presented in this book is based on the training and professional experience of the author. The treatments recommended in this book should not be undertaken without first consulting a physician. Proper laboratory and clinical monitoring is essential to achieving the goals of finding safe and natural treatments. This book was written for informational and educational purposes only. It is not intended to be used as medical advice.

To my father, Ellis. my first and best thyroid patient. I learned a tremendous amount from you.

And ,

To my family for all of their love and support, Allison, Hailey and Jessica,

To my staff: Thanks for your help and support,

And,

Of course, thanks to my patients. I am still learning from you every day.

Contents

Foreword

Having spent more than thirty years researching and working in the field of thyroid and other endocrine imbalances, I found Dr. Brownstein's book, **_Overcoming Thyroid Disorders,_** exciting and refreshing to read. Physicians were more adequately equipped to diagnose and treat thyroid disorders prior to the development of laboratory testing. At the turn of the 20th century, physicians were taught about the importance of a careful examination of the patient, and also to take into account the huge spectrum of factors that affect the vital balance of hormones, which in turn affects every cell in the body.

In modern medicine, the crucial role of the endocrine system has been lost, both in the literature and in the examination room. Twenty-first century medicine misses the importance of the clinical diagnosis as opposed to the laboratory diagnosis. For example, blood tests may only identify 2% to 5% of hypothyroid cases, often leaving many hypothyroid individuals classified as "normal" while their thyroid deficiency leaves them vulnerable to everything from heart disease to depression. We now have many hyperactive children on Ritalin whose actual problem is low thyroid. We now have depressed adults taking a pharmacopoeia of psychotropic drugs, many with serious side effects, treating symptoms and not the cause. Today, infertility clinics are filled with women who can't conceive, yet no one has ever properly evaluated their endocrine systems.

The literature clearly shows that prior to the reliance on blood tests for diagnosing hypothyroidism, nearly all infertile women, and those who suffered repeated miscarriages, were given natural thyroid hormone, and in most cases the infertility was resolved.

Broda O. Barnes, M.D., a pioneer in the field of thyroid and other hormonal disturbances, founded the Broda O. Barnes, MD Research Foundation, Inc. Dr. Barnes, being light-years ahead of his time, recognized that medicine was creating a nation of "paper physicians". Dr. Barnes was referring to physicians who relied solely on laboratory testing, often at the expense of the clinical picture.

David Brownstein, M.D., both in this book and in his practice, clearly understands how patients should be hormonally evaluated, diagnosed and treated. He does not rely solely on the laboratory testing for diagnosing, but takes into account the patient's clinical signs and symptoms, familial history, and includes all aspects of a patient's health. Dr. Brownstein impresses upon us not only the importance of hormones and their balance, but also how the endocrine system interacts with nutrients, lifestyle and the environment. Reading the case histories in this book shows us that Dr. Brownstein has truly resurrected the lost art of diagnosing. This, coupled with his kindness, and his sincere interest in his patients, has made him an extraordinary physician.

Overcoming Thyroid Disorders is an important work for those interested in hormonal aspects of health and general well being, both for physicians and their patients.

Patricia A. Puglio, President
BRODA O. BARNES, MD RESEARCH FOUNDATION, INC.
P.O. Box 110098
Trumbull, CT 06611
Phone 203-261-2101
Fax   203 261-3017
www.brodabarnes.org

Foreword to 2nd Edition

Overcoming Thyroid Disorders, 2nd Edition, is a continuum of the dedication, work, and heart, of David Brownstein, M.D. Dr. Brownstein is a physician who truly cares about his patients' health and well being. An inveterate researcher, Dr. Brownstein's quest for the truth has benefited his patients and colleagues with whom he is so willing to share his knowledge.

Broda O. Barnes, M.D., PhD, a researcher and pioneer in the field of thyroid and endocrine imbalances, stated in the 1960's that two things would forever change the face of properly diagnosing and treating hypothyroidism. The first development was the use of the blood test to diagnose hypothyroidism. The second development was the use of synthetic thyroid hormone to treat hypothyroidism.

Dr. Barnes' research pointed out that the blood tests would be inaccurate as thyroid hormone is not utilized in the blood, it is utilized in the cells of the body. Furthermore, his research proved that natural, desiccated thyroid hormone worked more efficiently in the body, and was more equivalent to the body's own endogenous production of thyroid hormone.

These two historical events have perplexed many in the medical profession, preventing some physicians from being able to help their patients. However, Dr. Brownstein's quest for knowledge and desire to explore the research and history in the field of thyroid disorders has given him the ability and resources to help many people who might otherwise have gone untreated. In addition, Dr. Brownstein, recognizing the importance of iodine in the body, has, in my opinion, become an expert in this field.

The Broda O. Barnes, M.D., Research Foundation, Inc. has had Dr. Brownstein lecture on the importance of iodine on several occasions, and each time the attending physicians are impressed with his knowledge and willingness to share this information. Dr. Brownstein also has an in-depth knowledge and understanding of the importance of a good diet and the nutritional supplementation necessary for proper endocrine function.

At the Broda O. Barnes, M.D. Research Foundation's 2007 Fall Endocrinology Conference, Richard Pooley, M.D. lectured on "Pioneers in Nutrition and Endocrinology". After hearing several of Dr. Brownstein's lectures, Dr. Pooley summed it up best when he told the audience he believed Dr. Brownstein to be one of our "modern day pioneers", putting him in the same realm as Broda O. Barnes, M.D., Jacques Hertoghe, M.D., and Eugene Hertoghe, M.D., our forefathers of endocrinology, and Dr. Weston A Price, a pioneer in nutrition. David Brownstein, M.D. has certainly earned this honor.

Patricia A. Puglio, President

BRODA O. BARNES, M.D. RESEARCH FOUNDATION, INC.

P.O. Box 110098

Trumbull, CT 06611

Phone: 203-261-2101

Fax: 203-261-3017

www.brodabarnes.org

January, 2008

Preface to 2nd Edition

It has been seven years since I wrote the book ***Overcoming Thyroid Disorders.*** It is hard to believe the book is seven years old. I have written this new edition to provide the reader with updated information on how to holistically treat thyroid disorders.

One of the most common questions my patients ask is, "Which thyroid medication is the best?" There is no "best" medication. This book was written to inform the reader that each patient is a unique biochemical individual. Therefore, each patient needs his/her own unique treatment plan. This book should provide you with a roadmap about which options are available in order to treat the underlying cause(s) of thyroid disorders.

Iodine is an integral nutrient for promoting thyroid function. Presently, iodine deficiency is occurring at epidemic levels. I will introduce the concept of using therapeutic doses of iodine to promote and maintain optimal thyroid function.

So often, conventional medicine does not search for or treat the underlying conditions of an illness. The most commonly used drug therapies primarily treat the symptoms of the illness rather than treating the underlying cause(s) of the illness. However, most of the commonly used drug therapies have numerous side effects associated with them.

A holistic approach, as outlined in this book, searches for the underlying cause(s) of the illness and then formulates a safe and effective natural treatment plan to help the body overcome the illness.

I have had a strong interest in thyroid disorders for over 15 years now. Solely relying on the conventional blood tests to make a diagnosis of a thyroid problem will result in a misdiagnosis in a large number of patients. These patients are subsequently diagnosed with other disorders such as depression or fibromyalgia. Many times, these patients are suffering from a hormonal imbalance, particularly a thyroid hormonal imbalance. Treating the underlying cause of the illness, in this case a thyroid disorder, is the correct action to take.

Finally, I wrote this book to give support to the patient suffering from a thyroid disorder. I wanted to provide you with hope and confidence in your quest to achieve your optimum health. In my practice, a holistic approach using safe and effective natural therapies has continually proven itself successful. This book was written to educate **you** to take charge of **your** own health care decisions.

TO ALL OF OUR HEALTH!

January, 2008

Chapter 1

Introduction

Introduction

This book will supply the reader with a road map to follow in order to reverse thyroid illness and help achieve optimum health. Unlike the conventional approach to illness, which revolves around the treatment of symptoms, the ideas outlined in this book involve searching for the underlying cause(s) of the illness and then formulating a holistic treatment plan. This holistic treatment program can include using natural hormones, vitamin and mineral supplementation, dietary changes and detoxification.

You will learn how a holistic program can be implemented in order to treat thyroid and other hormonal disorders primarily by using natural items. Chapter 2 discusses how to diagnose and treat hypothyroidism. I was trained both in medical school and in my residency that the proper way to diagnose thyroid problems was to rely primarily on the blood tests, particularly the TSH test. If the blood tests were normal, most likely, there was not a thyroid problem.

When I started practicing medicine, I often checked thyroid blood tests. If they were normal (as they often were), I told the patient that there was nothing wrong with their thyroid gland. If they were abnormal, I instituted treatment. I often ignored the patient's signs and symptoms if the lab tests were normal. Now, I am more convinced than ever that solely relying on the patient's blood tests without taking into account the physical exam as well as the patient's history will result in a misdiagnosis for many patients.

After finishing medical school and completing residency, I first became aware that perhaps the blood tests did not tell the whole story in evaluating thyroid problems. I was intrigued by the by the ideas offered by Broda O. Barnes, M.D. in his book, Hypothyroidism, the Unsuspected Illness (1976). Dr. Barnes wrote eloquently of his 50-year experience of treating hypothyroid individuals. Dr. Barnes was a pioneer in the treatment of thyroid disorders and throughout his career he maintained that the thyroid blood tests do not tell the whole story.

Dr. Barnes earned degrees in chemistry and biochemistry along with a PhD. in physiology of the thyroid gland. He was an Assistant Professor of Medicine at the University of Illinois. Dr. Barnes published over 100 research papers and authored four books about thyroid and other endocrine disorders. A non-profit foundation has been set up in his name, The Broda O. Barnes, M.D. Research Foundation. See Appendix B for more information on the Broda O. Barnes, M.D. Research Foundation.

Dr. Barnes pointed out that thyroid hormone exerts its influence on every cell in the body <u>inside</u> the cells while the blood tests only measure the circulating thyroid hormone levels <u>outside</u> the cells. Thirty years later, Dr. Barnes' comments about thyroid hormone tests are still valid.

One of Dr. Barnes' basic tenets was that if the thyroid gland was not properly balanced a wide variety of medical problems could develop. Oftentimes, the thyroid is not suspected as the culprit for many of these conditions, because the blood tests results are "within normal limits." Table 1 lists potential symptoms and diagnoses associated with thyroid and other hormonal imbalances.[1]

Table 1: Symptoms and Diagnoses of Thyroid and Other Endocrine Imbalances

Acne	Eczema	Low Immune System
Allergies	Endometriosis	Memory Impairment
Arthritis	Fatigue	Mental Disorders
Birth Defects	Fluid Retention	Muscle Loss
Brittle Nails	Gout	Muscle Weakness
Cancer	Hair Loss	Multiple Sclerosis
Candida	Headaches	Nervousness
Chronic Fatigue	Heart Palpitations	Nutritional Imbalances
Constipation	High Cholesterol	Overweight
Coronary Artery Disease	Hyperinsulinemia	P.M.S.
Cystic Breasts	Hypertension	Premature Aging
Cystic Ovaries	Infertility	Psoriasis
Decreased Sex Drive	Intolerance to Cold	Repeated Infections
Diabetes	Intolerance to Heat	Ridged Nails
Dry Skin	Low Blood Pressure	Underweight

Over 35 years ago, Dr. Barnes wrote, "Forty percent of the American people—four of every ten children and adults—today are suffering needlessly and many are dying for lack of an ingredient vital for health. Is the ingredient unknown? No. Or unavailable? No. For years, medicine has recognized the role of the deficiency in some areas of health and disease and has had clues to its great importance in many other areas. But the knowledge too often has not been used—and still is not being used—because of the unreliability of laboratory tests. [These laboratory tests] have failed to show the deficiency even when doctors could see its manifestations clearly enough in patients before them. And while laboratory tests have erred and have misled both doctors and patients, patients have suffered."[2] The 'ingredient' to which Dr. Barnes was referring is thyroid hormone. I believe that Dr. Barnes' ideas, written over 30 years ago, are still true today. In Chapter 2, I will discuss the inadequacy of relying solely on the thyroid laboratory tests.

Coronary Artery Disease and Hypothyroidism

Perhaps Dr. Barnes' most important and extensive research project dealt with coronary artery disease. Dr. Barnes reviewed over 70,000 autopsy records in order to compare the cause of deaths that occurred between 1930 and 1970 in Graz, Austria. Dr. Barnes found that in 1930, before the advent of antibiotics, most deaths were due to infections and these deaths occurred at a relatively young age, less than 50 years old. Deaths from heart attacks were rare. In 1930, infection was effectively killing off the weak at a young age.

By 1970, due to the use of antibiotics, infections were causing fewer deaths than in 1930. However, deaths from heart attacks increased 1,000 percent since 1930. Compared to 1930, in

1970 people were surviving to an older age and dying of a new cause—heart attacks. Dr. Barnes' hypothesis was that, "Either something new had entered the picture to cause the increase [in heart attacks], or those surviving premature deaths from infections were prone to develop heart disease. Careful study of the autopsy protocols indicated that the latter was true."[3]

The connection between the young individuals who died of infections in 1930 and the older individuals who died of heart attacks in 1970 was found in Dr. Barnes' research. The autopsy reports reviewed by Dr. Barnes showed that both groups, the young who died in 1930 and the old who died in 1970, had signs of advanced coronary artery disease. The only connection Dr. Barnes could draw to explain the cause of death in both groups was that both groups were suffering from the same problem: hypothyroidism.

After the advent of antibiotics, the hypothyroid population now began surviving infections and living to an older age. They began procreating, therefore creating new generations of hypothyroid individuals. As this group of people lived to an older age, now surviving infections through the use of antibiotics, the ravages of hypothyroidism began affecting them. This often took the form of coronary artery disease.

It is well known that the immune system does not function optimally in a hypothyroid individual, therefore increasing the risk of infection. The use of antibiotics often enables the hypothyroid individual to overcome the illness, as illustrated in Dr. Barnes' study. However, long-standing hypothyroidism, untreated over many years, will predispose the individual to developing coronary artery disease as well as other signs of hypothyroidism.

Coronary artery disease is the number one killer in this country. It has been the number one killer since antibiotics were introduced after World War II. Tens of millions of dollars have been spent studying why coronary artery disease affects such a wide range of the population. High cholesterol levels have been implicated as the cause of death due to heart disease. When patients see their doctors today it is customary to have their cholesterol level checked. If the cholesterol level is high, the physician is quick to prescribe a cholesterol-lowering drug. But, perhaps the elevated cholesterol is only a symptom of another problem: hypothyroidism.

It has been known for over 70 years that hypothyroidism predisposes one to have high cholesterol levels. If a diagnosis of high cholesterol is made, then a proper search for an underlying cause of the high cholesterol should be conducted.

I have treated numerous individuals diagnosed with high cholesterol levels diagnosed by other physicians. If there is an elevated cholesterol level present, then a thorough search for why there is a hypercholesterolemic situation should be undertaken. My clinical experience has clearly shown that many of these hypercholesterolemic patients are not suffering from a 'statin-deficiency situation'. I have found that a large percentage of individuals with elevated cholesterol levels have thyroid and other hormonal imbalances present. Correcting the hormonal imbalance(s) in these patients often times will correct the hypercholsterolemic problem without the use of a drug therapy. Chapter 7 will provide more information on this subject.

When the hormonal system is appropriately re-balanced, oftentimes the cholesterol level lowers dramatically. When one considers all of the possible signs of hypothyroidism (See Table 1, Pg. 22), the consequences of untreated and undiagnosed hypothyroidism are staggering.

After reading Dr. Barnes' book, I began to think about some of my patients who had chronic illnesses and were not responding well to medical therapy. One such patient was Ellis.

Ellis, age 61, had his first heart attack at age 41. He had his first coronary artery bypass surgery at age 48, and a second coronary artery bypass surgery at age 55. Angioplasty was performed at ages 58 and 60. Ellis suffered from continual angina for 18 years. He was diagnosed with high cholesterol levels, with a cholesterol level of 350ng/d, and the cholesterol level was unresponsive to any cholesterol-lowering medication. Although I counseled Ellis on dietary modifications, he refused to change his eating habits (much to my consternation). Ellis was overweight and he had a great deal of difficulty losing weight. After I read the book, **Hypothyroidism, the Unsuspected Illness**, by Dr. Barnes, I thought of Ellis. I called him into the office and told him I wanted to check a few things. When I checked Ellis' thyroid blood tests, his TSH level (see Chapter 2) was in the normal range. However, Ellis had low levels of the active thyroid hormone T3, as well as low basal body temperatures—96.7 degrees Fahrenheit (normal 97.8-98.2 degrees Fahrenheit). Furthermore, Ellis had many symptoms of hypothyroidism including: dry skin, weight gain, edema, poor nails, constipation, fatigue and hypertension. When I placed Ellis on a small amount of Armour® Thyroid and balanced the other hormones in his body (see Chapter 7), he made a dramatic recovery. Ellis' cholesterol fell dramatically to less than 200, without a change in his diet. Many of the other signs of hypothyroidism also dramatically improved including the fatigue, dry skin, hypertension and constipation. He also lost 25 pounds in a few months. In addition, his 18-year history of angina resolved one week after starting the thyroid hormone. Ellis' family and friends could all see the difference and people were asking him "What are you doing?," since he looked and acted so much better.

Ellis is one example of what undiagnosed and untreated hypothyroidism can do to an individual. I believe there are tens of thousands of people suffering needlessly from thyroid and other hormonal imbalances because laboratory tests are not sensitive enough. As physicians, we need to realize we are treating patients and not just laboratory tests. This book will explore this concept in more detail.

The case study on Ellis had a profound impact on the way I practiced medicine. Ellis was my father. Once I saw the change in my father's health I began to look at how hormonal imbalances, particularly thyroid hormone imbalances, impact one's health. Furthermore, I began to research ways of using natural approaches to help individuals overcome illness and achieve their optimal health. This book will illustrate some of those practices.

This book will give the reader a novel, holistic approach to diagnosing as well as treating thyroid disorders. A holistic approach treats more than just laboratory tests; it sets up a unique treatment program designed specifically for the individual patient. My holistic treatment plan for thyroid disorders involves looking not only at laboratory tests, but also at the physical exam signs, symptoms, diet, detoxification pathways, nutritional status and other pertinent information. In putting these various pieces of the puzzle together, a comprehensive, individualized plan can be undertaken to help the body recover from thyroid and other chronic disorders.

I have found excellent results by treating my patients with natural items, including bioidentical natural hormones, vitamins, minerals, herbs and diet. I have written this book to provide hope and present a holistic treatment plan for individuals trying to overcome thyroid and other chronic disorders.

[1] Adapted from Brodabarnes.org web site
[2] Barnes, Broda. Hypothyroidism, The Unsuspected Illness. Harper and Row. 1976. p. vii.
[3] Barnes, Broda. IBID. p. 160-161

Chapter 2

Hypothyroidism

Hypothyroidism

This Chapter will review the importance of maintaining adequate thyroid function, particularly in an under active thyroid state (i.e., hypothyroidism). The thyroid gland is a butterfly-shaped gland located in the lower part of the neck. Though it weighs less than an ounce, the thyroid gland is responsible for many critical functions in the body.

Every single muscle, organ and cell in the body depends on adequate thyroid hormone levels for achieving and maintaining optimal functioning. Thyroid hormone acts as the body's metabolic regulator. In a hypothyroid state, the thyroid gland is releasing inadequate amounts of thyroid hormone to meet the body's metabolic demands, and the metabolic rate is therefore reduced. In a hyperthyroid state, the thyroid gland is releasing excess amounts of thyroid hormone which results in an elevated metabolic rate. This Chapter will review the hypothyroid state. Chapter 5 will review the hyperthyroid condition.

The thyroid gland secretes approximately one teaspoon of thyroid hormone over an entire year. This teaspoon of thyroid hormone must drive the metabolic rate of every single cell in the body. Small variations in this amount will have wide ramifications on the health of the individual. It is impossible for the body to function at an optimum level of health if there is inadequate production of thyroid hormone.

What happens when the thyroid gland produces an inadequate amount of thyroid hormone? A constellation of symptoms develops. These symptoms are collectively referred to as hypothyroidism. Table 1 lists the signs and symptoms of hypothyroidism.

Table 1: Signs and Symptoms of Hypothyroidism

Brittle nails	Hypotension
Cold hands and feet	Inability to concentrate
Cold intolerance	Infertility
Constipation	Irritability
Depression	Menstrual Irregularities
Difficulty swallowing	Muscle Cramps
Dry skin	Muscle Weakness
Elevated Cholesterol	Nervousness
Essential Hypertension	Poor memory
Eyelid swelling	Puffy eyes
Fatigue	Slower heartbeat
Hair loss	Throat pain
Hoarseness	Weight Gain

How Common Is Hypothyroidism?

The prevalence of hypothyroidism is staggering. The Colorado Thyroid Disease Prevalence Study estimated that the rate of hypothyroidism in the general population was approximately 10%.[1] In the United States, this may mean that 13 million adults have an undiagnosed hypothyroid condition. Although this study used blood testing alone to diagnose a hypothyroid condition, my research has shown that relying solely on blood tests for this diagnosis will result in missing approximately 30% of those who have a hypothyroid condition. A holistic approach, which takes into account the laboratory tests, the basal body temperatures as well as the patient's signs and symptoms will identify many more individuals suffering from hypothyroidism. It is my opinion that the true figure for hypothyroidism is closer to 40% of the population or approximately 52 million adult Americans.

Thyroid Function

The thyroid gland produces 2 major hormones, Thyroxine (T4) and Triiodothyronine (T3) (see Figure 1). These two hormones work inside the cells of the body, primarily influencing the metabolism of the cells. In other words, thyroid hormone helps the cell machinery produce energy. When there is an adequate amount of thyroid hormone, the cell machinery functions normally and the metabolism of the cells (and the body) occurs at a normal level. When there is an inadequate amount of thyroid hormone produced (i.e., hypothyroidism), the metabolism of the cells (and the body) will decline, and the signs and symptoms of hypothyroidism will be present.

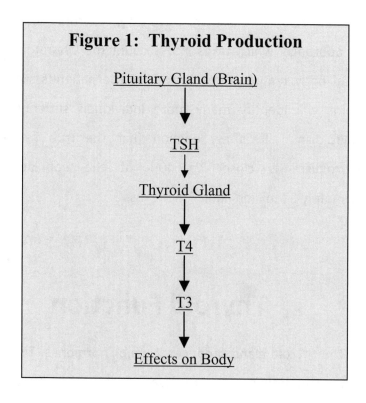

Figure 1: Thyroid Production

Pituitary Gland (Brain)

TSH

Thyroid Gland

T4

T3

Effects on Body

The thyroid produces much more T4 (approximately 80%) than T3 (approximately 20%). T3 is much more active than T4 (about 300% more active)[2] and T3 is the thyroid hormone that actually increases the metabolism inside the cells. The majority of T4 is actually converted into T3 inside the cells of the body.

How Is The Thyroid Gland Stimulated?

A pituitary hormone, known as Thyroid Stimulating Hormone or TSH (See Figure 1 above) stimulates the thyroid gland. When TSH is secreted from the pituitary gland, it causes the thyroid gland to release thyroid hormone. TSH is very sensitive to T4 and to T3. When the body has adequate amounts of thyroid hormone available, TSH levels are lowered so that the thyroid gland can lower its production of hormones.

How Is Hypothyroidism Diagnosed? The Conventional Approach

This section is divided into the **conventional** diagnosis and the **holistic** diagnosis of hypothyroidism. The **conventional** approach to diagnosing hypothyroidism primarily revolves around the measurement of thyroid blood tests, primarily the thyroid stimulating hormone (TSH) test.

If the TSH is elevated, it is a sign that the pituitary gland is sensing a low thyroid hormone level in the body, and the TSH is being secreted in order to stimulate the thyroid gland to produce more thyroid hormone.   If the TSH test is normal, many physicians believe that automatically rules out a hypothyroid state. See Figure 2 for TSH ranges.

Figure 2: TSH Ranges

TSH Normal Range: 0.4-4.5mIU/L
TSH Hypothyroid: > 4.5mIU/L

The Problems with the TSH Test

The TSH test has been the 'gold standard' in conventional medicine for diagnosing hypothyroidism for over 30 years. The normal range for the TSH test reported in most laboratories is from 0.5-4.5 mIU/L. When TSH values fall above this range (i.e.,

>4.5mIU/L), a diagnosis of hypothyroidism is given. This reference range was established to include 95% of the population. Therefore, 5% of the population, which falls outside of this reference range, should be classified as having a thyroid disorder.

However, as reported in the Colorado Thyroid Study (mentioned above), many researchers believe that the true incidence of hypothyroidism is significantly higher than 5%. Dr. AP Weetman, professor of medicine, wrote in the British Medical Journal, "Even within the reference range of around 0.5-4.5 mIU/L, a high thyroid stimulating hormone concentration (>2mIU/L) was associated with an increased risk of future hypothyroidism. The simplest explanation is that thyroid disease is so common that many people predisposed to thyroid failure are included in a laboratory's reference population, which raises the question whether thyroid replacement is adequate in patients with thyroid stimulating hormone levels above 2 mIU/L. The high frequency of overt and subclinical hypothyroidism observed raises another contentious issue--namely, whether screening for hypothyroidism is worthwhile."[3]

Therese Hertoghe, a Belgian endocrinologist also feels that the TSH test is not sensitive enough in identifying a hypothyroid condition. In Dr. Hertoghe's experience, the TSH test may only identify 2-5% of the hypothyroid individuals.[4] Dr. Hertoghe recommends correlating the blood test results with the clinical picture in order to secure an accurate diagnosis of hypothyroidism.

It has been my experience that relying solely on the TSH test will result in under-diagnosing many individuals who are suffering from hypothyroidism—up to 30% of the population. Dr. Barnes (recalled from Chapter 1) agreed that the laboratory tests should not be the sole judge of whether there is hypothyroidism present or not. He wrote, "...all commonly used lab tests for thyroid function leave much to be desired, that they are useful in some but not all cases, and that they are no substitute for a good physician's knowledge of what thyroid deficiency can bring about and his expert clinical impression of what it may be doing in the case of an individual patient."[5] Over 30 years ago, Dr. Barnes wrote about the inadequacies of solely relying upon laboratory tests in *Hypothyroidism, The Unsuspected Illness.*

Should the TSH 'Normal' Range be Changed?

There is great controversy in conventional medicine about where the 'normal' TSH range should be set. There are many physicians and organizations who believe the 'normal' upper limit of the TSH range should be lowered from 4.5mIU/l to 3mIU/l. This small change may result in a doubling of the numbers of individuals diagnosed as hypothyroid via blood tests—from approximately 13 million to 26 million individuals.

Figure 3: Proposed TSH Ranges

Present TSH 'Normal' Range (mIU/L)	Proposed TSH 'Normal' Range (mIU/L)
0.5-4.5	0.5-2.0

So, what should be the 'normal' TSH range? It is not an easy question to answer. It must be understood that the TSH test is only one measure of thyroid function. I do not think the TSH test should be used as the sole test, without regard to other lab tests, the physical exam as well as the history of the patient. Each patient is a unique biochemical individual. Some may do better at a TSH of 1.0mIU/L, while another may do better at a TSH of 3.0mIU/L. That is why it is so important to do a complete holistic workup (as outlined in this book) which includes looking at the rest of the thyroid blood tests as well as evaluating the nutritional status of the patient. Only with a complete holistic approach can you achieve the best results.

Having said that, my experience has shown that the vast majority of patients have optimal thyroid function when the TSH is between 0.3-2.0 mIU/L.

The Holistic Approach to Diagnosing Hypothyroidism

The **holistic** approach to diagnosing hypothyroidism is very different from the standard conventional model of relying only on the blood tests. I believe it is inappropriate to rely solely on laboratory tests to diagnose hypothyroidism, as this will miss many individuals suffering from this condition. A holistic approach includes looking at the following components:

1. Thyroid Blood tests
2. Medical history
3. Basal body temperatures
4. Physical exam

1. Thyroid Blood Tests

In my practice, I check thyroid blood tests and correlate them with the signs and symptoms as well as the basal body temperatures. This is a comprehensive, holistic approach to diagnosing hypothyroidism. As previously indicated, solely relying on the blood tests will miss many individuals suffering from hypothyroidism.

It is important to check more than just the TSH test. I have found it valuable to check T3 and T4 levels. If you recall from Figure 1 (p. 36), T3 is the active thyroid hormone that gets inside the cells and runs the metabolic machinery. TSH is more reflective of T4 levels. I have seen many patients who have normal T4 and TSH levels, but have low T3 levels, and therefore have many of the signs and symptoms of hypothyroidism. Solely relying on TSH testing will miss many of these hypothyroid individuals that have low T3 levels.

Poor T4 Converters

Many people do not adequately convert T4 into T3 and thus will be hypothyroid even though the TSH test falls within the normal range. I refer to these individuals as 'Poor T4 to T3 Converters'. Please see Figure 3 (page 44).

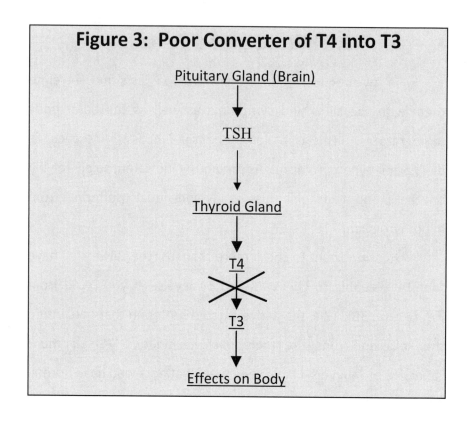

Figure 3: Poor Converter of T4 into T3

Pituitary Gland (Brain)

↓

TSH

↓

Thyroid Gland

↓

T4

T3

↓

Effects on Body

Because T4 levels are often maintained in these individuals the TSH test will often fall in the normal range. However, in many individuals, the more active form of thyroid hormone, T3, will be suppressed. Therefore, the 'Poor T4 to T3 Converter,' having a normal TSH, will exhibit many of the signs and symptoms of hypothyroidism. There are many reasons why an individual will not convert T4 into T3. Please see Table 2 (page 45). More information on T4 to T3 conversion problems will be found in Chapter 3.

Table 2: Factors That Cause an Inability to Convert T4 to T3

Nutrient Deficiencies	Medications	Other
Chromium	Beta Blockers	Aging
Copper	Birth Control Pills	Alcohol
Iodine	Estrogen	Lipoic Acid
Iron	Iodinated Contrast Agents	Diabetes
Selenium	Lithium	Fluoride
Zinc	Phenytoin	Lead
Vitamin A	Steroids	Mercury
Vitamin B2	Theophylline	Obesity
Vitamin B6		Pesticides
Vitamin B12	**Diet**	Radiation
	Cruciferous Vegetables	Stress
	Soy	Surgery

Martha, a 58-year-old accountant had not felt well for 10 years. "I was o.k. until I hit menopause. Then, my life changed. I became extremely fatigued and I gained 20 pounds that I could not explain. It took my doctor six months to figure out that I had become hypothyroid," she said. Martha was treated with Synthroid, a synthetic T4 form of thyroid hormone, but she did not feel any better. She claimed, "When I started the Synthroid®, I thought I would feel better. But it didn't do much for me. I still have the weight and I am still tired." Also, she was always cold. Martha had cold hands and feet and she complained of having very dry skin. When I checked Martha's blood tests, her results were:

TSH 3.0 (normal 0.5-4.5 mU/l)

T4 148 (normal 80-180ug/dl)

T3 54 (normal 55-120ng/dl)

Examination of Martha's thyroid blood tests revealed an adequate production of T4 and normal TSH levels. However, Martha's T3 levels were on the low side, indicating a poor T4 to T3 conversion problem. Further examination of Martha revealed deficiencies of B Vitamins and protein. Her nutritional deficiencies were corrected by increasing her protein intake and adding B vitamins. In addition, I recommended that she replace Synthroid® (a T4 medication), with Armour® Thyroid. Armour® Thyroid contains T4 in addition to T3 and other substances that help the body convert T4 into the more active T3 thyroid hormone. (More information on thyroid medication can be found later in this chapter). After six weeks of this treatment regimen, all of Martha's hypothyroid symptoms improved. "It was like I woke up. My skin began to feel better and I began to feel better. Even my friends kept asking me what I was doing since I looked so much better," she exclaimed. Martha's lab tests revealed an improved *conversion of T4 to T3 (T4 150 ug/dl and T3 98 ng/dl).*

Martha's positive response from changing thyroid hormone medication and correcting nutritional imbalances is common. Many of my patients who were previously on T4 medications such as Synthroid® show significant improvement in their condition once they are switched to a more active thyroid hormone. The holistic approach for optimizing thyroid function involves taking into account the patient's history, a physical exam and basal body temperatures, and correlating these findings with the lab tests. This method is an effective, comprehensive treatment strategy for individuals with thyroid problems.

2. Medical History

When evaluating patients for thyroid problems, I initially take a history from them and do a physical exam. As seen in Table 2 (page 45), the manifestations of hypothyroidism are vast. Remember that thyroid hormone affects every cell in the body from the head to the toes. Therefore, underproduction of thyroid hormone will result in many different signs and symptoms throughout the entire body.

3. Basal Body Temperatures

As previously mentioned, one of the thyroid's main functions is to regulate the metabolism of every cell in the body. When adequate amounts of thyroid hormone are produced, the metabolic machinery inside each of the billions of cells runs at a normal pace. One by-product of this metabolic machinery is heat. The production of heat helps keep the body warm on cold days. However, in a hypothyroid condition, the metabolism of the cells runs at a much slower pace. Hypothyroid individuals will often complain of feeling cold much of the time, including having cold hands and feet. In fact, when the thyroid gland is removed from an otherwise normal animal, all metabolic activity in that animal is reduced.[6]

Maintaining a steady body temperature is one of the most crucial functions of the thyroid gland. Many of the enzymes, vitamins, minerals and chemical reactions that are utilized in the body are temperature sensitive. When the body temperature is maintained within a normal range, from 97.8-98.2 degrees Fahrenheit, the enzymes, vitamins, minerals and chemical reactions optimally function. Small variations in temperature, either elevated or depressed, will significantly decrease the utilization of these items.

How can you accurately measure this metabolic activity? This is a very difficult task. For over 50 years, physicians have been trying to develop a laboratory test that will actually measure the metabolism of the body. First, they relied on the Basal Metabolism Test, which proved inaccurate. Next, they relied on the protein-bound iodine test (i.e., PBI), which also failed. Finally, the thyroid hormone tests, T4 and TSH were touted as the 'gold standard' for diagnosing/monitoring thyroid function. At some point in time, each of these tests was accepted by the medical establishment as the optimal test of thyroid function. Over time, as the tests have been found to be inaccurate, it was determined that each test was missing many people who were suffering from hypothyroidism.

Now, the TSH test exists as the newest, best test. In my opinion, since we cannot measure the amount of thyroid hormone inside each of the billions of cells in the body, each test can provide some information, but should not be used solely to confirm or deny a diagnosis of hypothyroidism. To do so ensures missing many individuals who may be suffering from the ravages of hypothyroidism.

Basal Body Temperature Testing

One test that is underutilized is checking the basal temperature. When the thyroid is producing adequate amounts of thyroid hormone and the cells are able to utilize the thyroid hormone, the cells of the body are producing enough heat to

49

maintain a steady and normal body temperature (97.8-98.2 degrees Fahrenheit). The basal body temperature is best measured in the morning, upon awakening. I recommend using axillary (under the arm pit) temperatures. See Figure 4 for instructions on how to measure your basal body temperature. It is best to do the basal temperatures on consecutive days. Menstruating women need to do their basal temperatures at the beginning of their menstrual cycle, as outlined in Figure 4.

Figure 4: How to Measure the Basal Body Temperature

1. Shake down a basal thermometer the night before and place at your bedside or use a digital basal thermometer.

2. Upon awakening, place the thermometer snugly in your armpit for a period of 10 minutes and record your temperature for 5 days in a row. You must not get out of bed before checking your temperature or you will have an altered reading.

3. For women who are menstruating, the temperature should be taken starting on the second day of menstruation. This is the best time in a woman's menstrual cycle to get an accurate basal temperature. For men and postmenopausal women, it makes no difference when the temperatures are taken.

4. If your thyroid function is normal, your temperature should be in the range of 97.8-98.2 degrees Fahrenheit. A temperature below this may indicate a hypothyroid state.

5. You can also check oral or rectal temperatures. Normal oral/rectal temperatures should be in the range of 98.8-99.2 degrees Fahrenheit.

---

4. Physical Exam Signs

One of the most common findings I see in patients who suffer from hypothyroidism is poor eyebrow growth, especially the outer third of the eyebrows. This sign is known as the 'Sign of Hertoghe.'

Also, periorbital edema, or swelling under the eyes is another common finding in hypothyroid individuals. This condition has been described for almost 100 years in hypothyroid individuals. There are many other signs of hypothyroidism that can commonly be seen in a hypothyroid individual if they are looked for.

Katie, age 54, suffered from severe fatigue for six years. "I go to bed tired, and I wake up tired," she lamented. Also, Katie complained of other symptoms of hypothyroidism. She said, "I can't believe how I look. I feel like someone took a bicycle pump and blew up my face. Also, my hair is falling out and my skin is extremely dry no matter what I do to it." Katie's blood tests revealed significantly elevated TSH and a very low T3 level, indicating a hypothyroid condition. Within two months of treatment with Armour® Thyroid, many of Katie's symptoms were markedly better. "Even my friends were commenting how much better I looked. They all noticed that I looked like I had lost weight. I did lose a few pounds, but I think they were noticing the difference in my face. It no longer looks swollen," she said. Katie also reported a return of her energy level when the hypothyroidism was appropriately treated. Katie sent me a 'before and after' thyroid hormone picture of her face, where the difference in the puffiness of her face can clearly be seen. I have used these pictures to educate physicians and others about how an individual's face can look when they are suffering from hypothyroidism.

A Comprehensive Holistic Approach to Diagnosing Hypothyroidism

As previously stated, my clinical experience has shown that relying solely on the blood tests to diagnose hypothyroidism will miss many hypothyroid individuals. A more complete evaluation of the thyroid gland can be accomplished by using the blood tests in combination with the physical exam signs, the medical history and the basal body temperatures. This is truly a comprehensive holistic way to diagnose an individual with a complicated illness such as hypothyroidism. Relying solely on laboratory tests ignores the basic tenets of being a physician and treating the patient as an entire being.

Treatment of Hypothyroidism

The treatment of hypothyroidism varies greatly. I will divide this section into the **conventional treatment** and the **holistic treatment** of hypothyroidism.

CONVENTIONAL TREATMENT OF HYPOTHYROIDISM

The conventional treatment of hypothyroidism relies primarily on using synthetic derivatives of T4, Levothyroxine Sodium, more commonly known as Synthroid®, Levothroid®, Unithroid®, etc.

As previously mentioned, most conventional physicians will solely monitor TSH levels in order to gauge the functioning of the thyroid gland. TSH is very sensitive to circulating T4 levels. As T4 levels decline, TSH will increase, trying to stimulate the thyroid gland. As T4 levels increase, TSH levels will decline.

The problem with monitoring TSH levels is that it does not tell you how much T4 is converting to T3, the more active thyroid hormone. As previously mentioned, there is no lab test that can assess how T3 is functioning inside each of the billions of cells in the body. Relying solely on T4 monitoring and T4 treatment (i.e., Levothyroxine Sodium products--Synthroid®, Levothroid®, Unithroid®, etc.) will miss many of the cases of hypothyroidism and result in sub-optimal treatment for the condition.

HOLISTIC TREATMENT OF HYPOTHYROIDISM

The holistic approach to treating hypothyroidism is to look at the entire pathway shown in Figure 1 (page 36) and try to optimize thyroid function. As previously mentioned, many items interfere with the normal conversion of thyroid hormone from its inactive (T4) to its more active (T3) form (see Table 2 p. 45). Whether the treatment involves stopping drugs such as birth control pills or synthetic estrogens, correcting vitamin and nutrient deficiencies or using dietary strategies, the focus should be on maximizing the body's own thyroid production and utilization.

When medication is needed to treat hypothyroidism, I believe that using a desiccated glandular thyroid products (e.g., Armour® Thyroid, Nature-Thyroid™ or Westhroid™) are much more effective treatment options as compared to using T4 derivatives. My clinical experience with using desiccated thyroid has shown that it is a superior product as compared to the synthetic versions of thyroid hormone presently available (such as Synthroid® or Levothroid®). My experience parallels Dr. Barnes' conclusions from 30 years ago. In commenting on the experts of that time who recommended that only T4 was necessary to treat thyroid deficiency, Dr. Barnes wrote, "My results, on thousands of cases seen over a period of 43 years do not bear out their enthusiasm" for using only T4 products. "The discrepancy may be due to the fact that failures in therapeutic results have a habit of congregating in my office."[7]

Desiccated (i.e., heat dried) thyroid glandular products mentioned above are porcine (pig) derivative. Although it is not a direct duplicate of our own thyroid production (since it is porcine derived), it is the closest version we presently have available. Desiccated thyroid has T4 (like Synthroid®) but also has the more active thyroid hormone T3 and other factors that allow its conversion to T3 to take place more readily in the body. Table 3 compares desiccated thyroid to the synthetic thyroid versions currently available.

Table 3: Comparison of Contents of Desiccated Thyroid versus Synthetic Thyroid Hormones

Desiccated Thyroid	Levothyroxine Sodium
T4	T4
T3	
T2	
T1	
Calcitonin	
Selenium	
Diuretic Effect	

Beth, age 33, was unable to conceive. "I have been trying to have a baby for the last 3 years. My doctors cannot tell me why I cannot get pregnant," she said. Beth suffered with many of the signs of hypothyroidism including: cold extremities, hair loss, fatigue, PMS and dry skin. Beth had been taking Synthroid® for four years, but it was not helping her symptoms. Beth's blood tests indicated that she had an inability to convert T4 to T3 (T4 conversion block see page 43). When I changed Beth's thyroid replacement to Armour® Thyroid, all of her symptoms improved within four weeks. More importantly, Beth became pregnant two months later. She commented, "I was ecstatic. I couldn't believe how much better I felt with the Armour® Thyroid." I had not seen Beth for three years when she came to the office for a check up. After the birth of her child, Beth went to a physician who told her that Synthroid® was a better drug than Armour® Thyroid. He *claimed that Synthroid® was newer and it was more consistent as compared to Armour® Thyroid. After changing to Synthroid®, Beth wanted another child, but found she was again unable to conceive and she had many hypothyroid symptoms return. When I changed her thyroid back to Armour® Thyroid, she became pregnant six weeks later and again the hypothyroid symptoms resolved. "I will never go off the Armour® Thyroid again. I don't know how a doctor can tell **me** which thyroid pill is the best. **I can tell** which one works better for me. It is definitely the Armour® Thyroid."*

The relationship between infertility and hypothyroidism has been known for over 50 years. I have found many women with undiagnosed infertility problems actually have a hypothyroid condition. When the hypothyroid condition is properly treated, many times the infertility problem resolves.

Desiccated thyroid may also contain an unknown hormone that gives it an additional benefit. This unknown hormone may be a diuretic hormone, which is separate from the other hormones in Armour® (i.e., T4 and T3). Dr. Barnes was the first to propose this idea when he wrote, "Evidence suggests that a diuretic fraction [in Armour® Thyroid] may be present."[8] Levothyroxine sodium products (Synthroid®, Levothroid®, Unithroid®, etc.) do not have the diuretic effect that Armour® Thyroid has. This diuretic component of Armour® Thyroid helps to relieve the edema that is commonly found in hypothyroidism.

Thyroid production is very complex in the body. In addition to the production of T3 and T4 thyroid hormones, there are other thyroid hormones released from the thyroid gland, including T2 and T1 thyroid hormone. T2 hormone has been shown to help increase the metabolic rate, especially for muscles and fat tissue.[9] [10] I believe the added agents in a desiccated preparation such as Armour® Thyroid or Nature-Throid™ make it a much more useful product than the commonly prescribed synthetic versions (i.e., Synthroid®, Levothroid®, Unithroid®, etc). More importantly, I have observed much better clinical results in my patients with using desiccated thyroid (i.e., Armour® Thyroid) versus levothyroxine sodium products.

Some physicians feel that T3, being the more active thyroid hormone, provides the best results when treating hypothyroidism. Although I have had patients improve their condition with T3, I have not had the sustained success with treating hypothyroidism when using T3 as I have when using desiccated thyroid. Furthermore, T3 can be dangerous if the amounts used are too high or if used in individuals with hypoadrenal or cardiac problems. This will be explained in more detail in Chapter 5. However, small amounts of T3 added to T4 preparations do provide benefit in many individuals. A study from the *New England Journal of Medicine* found that adding a small amount of T3 to patients already being treated with T4 preparations (i.e., Synthroid®, Levothroid®, etc.) significantly improved mood and brain function.[11]

I see many patients in my practice that were diagnosed with hypothyroidism by another physician and placed on a levothyroxine sodium product such as Synthroid®. Although their blood tests improved with the use of Synthroid®, many of their symptoms did not improve. Upon changing their thyroid hormone to the desiccated version (i.e., Armour® Thyroid, Nature-Throid™, Westhroid™), their symptoms dramatically improve. I believe this improvement occurs because the body is able to convert the desiccated thyroid hormone (i.e., Armour® Thyroid) to the active hormone more efficiently. The next two case studies will illustrate why a desiccated thyroid hormone is much more effective than levothyroxine derivatives such as Synthroid®.

Louise, age 64, was diagnosed with hypothyroidism three years ago. "For five years I would tell my doctor that I was very fatigued. The fatigue became much worse, and I eventually had to quit my job. I gained 20 pounds, my hair began falling out and I had constant muscle aches and pains," she said. Louise was found to have an elevated TSH 30 mIU/l (Normal 0.5-4.5 mIU/l). She was treated with Synthroid®. She claimed, "I never felt much better with the Synthroid®. I kept telling my doctor that I was still tired, but he told me my blood tests (TSH) were normal on the Synthroid®. When I asked him, 'How come I am still tired?' he told me it must be depression. Now I know I don't feel well, but I am

not depressed." When I changed Louise's medication to Armour®
Thyroid, she noticed an immediate improvement. "It was like
night and day. I started to regain my energy and it was easier to
lose the weight. After two months of taking Armour® Thyroid, I
began to feel like my old self," she claimed. Louise's friends began
asking her what she was doing since she looked and acted so well.
"I just told my friends that I finally had my thyroid hormone
working. Now, they all want their thyroid levels checked," she
said.

Ken, age 35, was diagnosed with chronic fatigue
syndrome five years ago. An avid athlete, Ken had to give up all
sports. "Whenever I exerted myself, I felt awful. My body could
not recover from any physical activity," he claimed. Ken was
diagnosed with hypothyroidism two years ago and treated with
Levothroid® (a levothyroxine sodium product). He said, "It didn't
do a thing for me. I might as well have been taking a sugar pill."
When I examined Ken, he had many of the clinical signs of
hypothyroidism, including dry skin, puffiness under his eyes,
thickened tongue and very slow reflexes, even though he was
being treated with synthetic thyroid hormone. Ken's blood work
and basal body temperatures initially (while taking synthetic
thyroid hormone) were:

TSH 3.5miU/l (normal 0.2-4.7mIU/l)

T4 level was 98ug/dl (normal 5.0-12 ug/dl)
T3 level was low—56ng/dl (normal 55-160 ng/dl)
Basal Body Temperature average 96.6 degrees
Fahrenheit

Ken's blood tests revealed a T4 conversion problem (see Chapter 3) that was not being adequately addressed with the use of T4 preparations like Levothroid. Ken was switched to Armour® Thyroid and began to feel better within four weeks. "The change was dramatic. My energy began to return, I could think clearly, and I finally became able to do light exercise. I feel like I have been given my life back," he said. Ken's blood work also improved:

TSH 1.5 mU/l
T4 90 ug/d
T3 86 ng/dl

Why Don't Most Doctors Prescribe Desiccated Thyroid?

This section will deal with the question of why most physicians are reluctant to prescribe desiccated thyroid when there is a hypothyroid condition. One of the first things I learned in medical school was to use only levothyroxine sodium products (i.e., Synthroid®, Levothroid®, etc.) for treating thyroid problems. I was told that these products were the 'newest' and the 'best' products on the market. Furthermore, I was told that desiccated thyroid hormone, like Armour® Thyroid, was not consistent from dose to dose. In other words, each 30mg dose of Armour® Thyroid may or may not contain 30mg of Armour® Thyroid.

I do not know the origin of the complaint that desiccated thyroid is not consistent from dose to dose. The FDA has been aware of the poor consistency of some levothyroxine products for a number of years however there is no such concern with desiccated thyroid. In 1997, the FDA reported that "…no currently marketed orally administered levothyroxine sodium product has been shown to demonstrate consistent potency and stability and, thus, no currently marketed orally administered levothyroxine sodium product is generally recognized as safe and effective."[12] The FDA also wrote that Synthroid® has a long history of quality-control problems. Recently, two levothyroxine sodium drugs have received FDA approval for potency and consistency of their products—Levothroid® and Unithroid®.

I have not found a consistency problem with desiccated thyroid products. Because of the T4 conversion problem (see Chapter 3), a thyroid product that enhances the conversion of inactive (T4) to active (T3) thyroid hormone is bound to have a greater efficacy. In my experience, desiccated thyroid does have a more superior therapeutic effect than levothyroxine sodium products.

What other Brands of Thyroid Hormone are Available?

Armour® Thyroid contains some inactive ingredients (i.e., fillers) including cornstarch. People with allergies to cornstarch and the other fillers may have problems with Armour® Thyroid. There are other versions of thyroid hormone available on the market. Chapter 4 will review the different brands of thyroid hormone currently available.

Other versions of desiccated thyroid hormone include Westhroid™ and Nature-Throid™. Westhroid™, like Armour® Thyroid, is made from porcine thyroid glands. It also has a cornstarch binder in it. Nature-Throid™ is bound by microcrystalline cellulose, which is derived from paper. I have seen good responses from my patients with these two products. More about these products can be found in Chapter 4.

Final Thoughts

My clinical experience has clearly shown that using a more active form of thyroid hormone is almost always more effective than using T4 derivatives. As the body ages, the conversion of T4 to T3 declines and supporting this conversion process with nutrients and a more active thyroid hormone makes common sense. More importantly, patients feel better when given the proper thyroid hormone supplement for their condition.

In evaluating individuals with chronic illnesses, physicians must keep in mind that we are not treating laboratory tests. We are treating complex individuals who have differing presentations of their illnesses. We must use the safest, most effective treatment options available. For thyroid patients, I have found that ensuring that the body's conversion of T4 to T3 is optimal will improve the overall health of the patients as well as improve any chronic conditions.

[1] Canaris, Gay, et al. The Colorado Thyroid Disease Prevalence Study. Arch. Intern. Med. Vol 160, Feb 28, 2000

[2] Harrison's Principles of Internal Medicine. 14th Edition. 1998

[3] Weetman, A.P. "Fortnightly review: Hypothyroidism: screening and subclinical disease." British Medical Journal. 1997;314:1175 919 April

[4] Hertoghe, Therese. From lecture at Broda O. Barnes M.D. Research Foundation, Stamford CT, February, 2002

[5] Barnes, Broda. Hypothyroidism, The Unsuspected Illness. Harper and Row. 1976. p. 137

[6] Barnes, Broda. Hypothyroidism, The Unsuspected Illness. Harper and Row. 1976. p. 19

[7] Barnes, Broda. Is There a Third Hormone in the Thyroid Gland? Which Preparation Should be Used for Treatment? Journal of IAPM, Nov. 1982

[8] Barnes, Broda. Is There a Third Hormone in the Thyroid Gland? Which Preparation Should be Used for Treatment? Journal of IAPM, Nov. 1982

[9] Lanni, A, et al. Calorigenic effect of di-iodothyroidines in the rat. J. Physiol (Lond) 1996;494:831-37

[10] Horst, C., et al. Rapid stimulation of hepatic oxygen consumption by 3,5-di-iodo-l-thyrooninne. Biochem J. 1989;261:945-950

[11] Bunevicius, B., et al. Effects of thyroxine as compared with thyroxine plus triiodothyronine in patients with hypothyroidism. NEJM. 1999;340:424-429.

[12] Federal Register, August 14, 1997 (Vol. 62, Num 157)

Chapter 3

Poor T4 Converters and Thyroid Hormone Resistance

Poor T4 Converters and Thyroid Hormone Resistance

In Chapter 2, it was established that many individuals do not convert some, most, or all of the relatively inactive form of thyroid hormone-T4 to its more active hormone-T3. Thyroid hormone resistance is another condition that is responsible for causing much of the hypothyroidism that is present today. Thyroid hormone resistance can occur with an adequate production of thyroid hormone. In this case, there is resistance at the cellular level to thyroid hormone. It is very common to have normal thyroid blood tests when thyroid hormone resistance occurs. Thyroid hormone resistance is analogous to insulin resistance found in adult onset diabetes. This Chapter will explore thyroid hormone resistance and poor T4 converters in detail and describe why hypothyroidism is so prevalent today.

What is a 'Poor T4 Converter'?

In order to understand why there is so much hypothyroidism in the world today, one must understand how the thyroid works. The thyroid gland secretes T4 (or L-thyroxine) in response to the body's needs for thyroid hormone. T4 is a relatively inactive form of thyroid hormone. For T4 to effectively stimulate metabolism in the body, it must first be converted to T3, the active form of thyroid hormone. This conversion of T4 to T3 occurs in the organs of the body such as the kidneys, liver, brain, etc, by an enzyme called iodothyronine 5'deiodinase. When this conversion is not taking place at adequate levels, signs of hypothyroidism will be present. Figure 1 illustrates this concept.

Although both T4 and T3 are active thyroid hormones, T3 is much more active than T4. T3 is approximately three times more potent than T4.[1] It is T3 that is largely responsible for the effects of thyroid hormone on the metabolism of the body, such as producing heat, growing hair, etc.

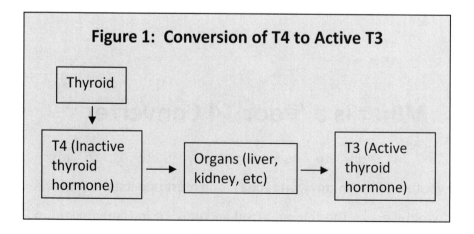

Figure 1: Conversion of T4 to Active T3

Thyroid

T4 (Inactive thyroid hormone) → Organs (liver, kidney, etc) → T3 (Active thyroid hormone)

In examining Figure 1, it becomes apparent that the optimal situation is when the body is able to convert as much T4 as possible into the more active thyroid hormone T3. If the body is unable to convert some, most, or all of T4 into T3, signs and symptoms of hypothyroidism will be observed. Also, any condition that impairs the production of T4 hormone will impact the production of the active T3 hormone as well. These situations can result in the manifestation of the signs of hypothyroidism, including cold extremities, a slower metabolism and other symptoms. Please see Chapter 2 for more information about hypothyroidism.

There are multiple factors that can result in a decrease of the conversion of T4 into T3. Some agents (i.e., certain drugs, nutritional deficiencies) can block this conversion. Other drugs may cause the T4 to be bound up by proteins in the blood stream. In addition other agents may cause a decrease in the production of T4 from the thyroid gland and will ultimately cause a decrease in the active thyroid hormone T3. In any of the above examples, the end result is a hypothyroid condition. Figure 2 illustrates the concept of a poor T4 to T3 converter.

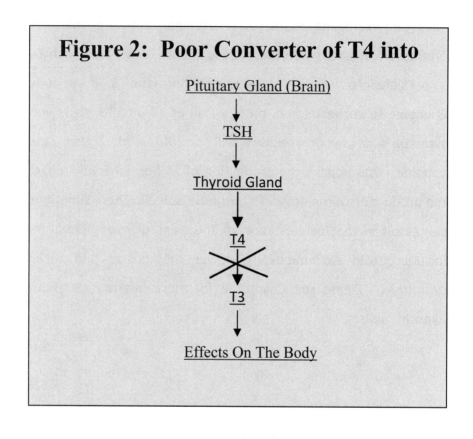

Figure 2: Poor Converter of T4 into

Pituitary Gland (Brain)

TSH

Thyroid Gland

T4

T3

Effects On The Body

The Problem with the TSH Test

Conventional medicine primarily relies on the TSH blood test to diagnose hypothyroidism. Chapter 2 explored this concept in more detail. The treatment of hypothyroidism in conventional medicine primarily revolves around the use of T4 products (i.e., Synthroid®, Levothroid®, Unithroid®).

The TSH test is very sensitive to T4. In fact, if T4 levels become elevated, TSH levels will fall. Therefore, when using laboratory values to diagnose hypothyroidism, the patients with elevated TSH tests are primarily treated with T4 products to lower the TSH values. However, if the body is unable to convert the inactive T4 to the active T3, many symptoms of hypothyroidism can still be present event though the blood test (i.e., TSH) can be normal. Dr. Kenneth Blanchard, an endocrinologist, agrees. "What doctors are always told is that the TSH test always gives a yes or no answer. In fact, I think this is fundamentally wrong. The pituitary TSH is controlled, not just by how much T4 and T3 are in circulation, but {by how much} T4 is converted into T3," he claims.[2]

Therefore, relying solely on the TSH test to monitor thyroid function may not give the whole picture of what is happening with thyroid function. People can still have the signs and symptoms of hypothyroidism (including low T3 levels), yet have normal T4 and TSH levels.

Tina, a 29-year-old woman from Amarillo, Texas, wrote me a letter about her experience with hypothyroidism.

Dear Dr. Brownstein,

I have been dealing with hypothyroidism for 12 years. I have been on Synthroid and other synthetic forms of thyroid hormone, with no luck. It has really started affecting me in the past year: losing hair, constipation, constantly tired, sluggishness, headaches, and mood swings.

*I started investing time into finding another solution and that is when I stumbled upon your book, **The Miracle of Natural Hormones, 3rd Edition.** With book in hand, I went to my doctor and suggested Armour® thyroid instead of Synthroid®.*

My doctor told me it would not help because my thyroid tests were normal. He said that I must have been imagining these disorders. He also commented that Armour® thyroid was the 'old way' of treating hypothyroidism and he refused to prescribe it.

I insisted on trying Armour® thyroid until he gave in. I have been taking Armour® thyroid for three months now and there is a HUGE difference. So much so, that my family notices! All of my symptoms are gone and my life is back.

If I did not read Dr. Brownstein's book, I would be asleep right now and I would not care about anything. Thank you Dr. Brownstein!

Tina's story illustrates the fallacy of simply following the blood tests to monitor a hypothyroid condition. Tina probably was not converting T4 into T3, thus exhibiting many of the signs of hypothyroidism even while taking T4 replacement (Synthroid®). Simply adjusting her thyroid medication to a more active form of thyroid hormone (Armour® thyroid) resulted in marked improvement in all of her hypothyroid symptoms. I have seen Tina's story repeat itself over and over again in my practice.

Factors that Inhibit the Conversion of T4 to T3

The conversion of T4 to T3 can be inhibited by many factors, as previously discussed in Chapter 2 (page 45). Table 1 (next page) lists other factors that cause an inability to convert T4 into T3. There are several ways this can occur. The enzyme, 5'-deiodinase (5'D-I), is responsible for the conversion of T4 into the more active thyroid hormone T3. This enzyme can malfunction when there are nutritional deficiencies, which can lead to mineral imbalances (particularly zinc and selenium). Also, some drugs can cause T4 to be bound up in the serum, making it less available for the conversion to T3. Either way, this will lead to less T4 being converted to T3, and give the clinical picture of hypothyroidism. For purposes of this book, all such factors that lessen the conversion of T4 into T3 will be referred to as 'poor T4 converters.'

Because so many different agents (drugs, illness, trauma, aging, etc.) can block the conversion of T4 to T3, caution must be taken when evaluating thyroid blood tests. Physicians need to be aware that the blood tests alone may not tell the whole story. I have seen many patients whose thyroid blood tests (TSH and T4 tests) were normal, yet there were very low levels of T3 present. Appropriate treatment designed to improve their conversion of thyroid hormone, along with therapeutic doses of desiccated thyroid hormone, significantly improved their condition. Their recoveries were reflected in improved T3 levels and, more importantly, an improvement in their condition.

Table 1: Factors Associated with Decreased T4 to T3 Conversion

Alpha-Lipoic Acid
Anti TPO antibodies
Chronic illness
Cigarette smoking
Drugs (propylthiouracil, methimazole,dexamethasone, propranolol, amiodarone, birth control pills, estrogens, lithium)
External radiation
Fasting
Growth hormone deficiency
Heavy metal toxicity including mercury toxicity
Hemochromatosis
High stress
Iodinated cholestographic agents (used in x-ray procedures)
Low adrenal states
Malnutrition
Mineral and vitamin deficiencies (selenium, Vitamin A, Vitamin B6 and Vitamin B12)
Old age
Physical trauma
Postoperative state
Soy

Factors Associated With a Decreased T4 to T3 Conversion

As illustrated in Table 1, there are numerous factors associated with a decreased conversion of inactive thyroid hormone (T4) to active thyroid hormone (T3). This section will explore many of these items.

Old age

In the elderly, researchers have noted a decrease in the conversion of T4 to T3.[3] [4] Some researchers believe this decrease is due to mineral deficiencies that occur more commonly in the elderly, including selenium deficiency.[5]

Malnutrition

In the malnourished state, the body becomes deficient in various vitamins and minerals. The enzyme responsible for converting T4 to T3 is very sensitive to selenium and zinc status. Deficiencies in either of these items, as found in malnourished states, will result in a poor T4 to T3 conversion, and lead to hypothyroid symptoms.

Also, poor protein intake will diminish the production of thyroid hormone.

Chronic illness

Chronic illness can cause alterations in thyroid hormones resulting in a hypothyroid state. Not everyone with a chronic illness will develop thyroid problems, but the longer and the more severe the illness, the more likely that thyroid dysfunction will become apparent.

Drugs

Many drugs alter thyroid production or the body's utilization of thyroid hormones. Drugs can interfere with thyroid function in a number of ways including:

1. Blocking the enzyme that converts T4 to T3
2. Decreasing the production of thyroid hormones
3. Blocking thyroid hormone at its receptor
4. Causing thyroid hormone to be bound in the blood by protein

There are many drugs that may negatively impact the thyroid gland resulting in a hypothyroid state. These include:

A. Birth control pills

Birth control pills contain estrogens. These estrogens, when taken orally, are responsible for increasing a protein (thyroxine binding globulin--TBG) that will effectively decrease the amount of thyroid hormone that is available for the body to use. This can lead to a hypothyroid state. I have successfully treated numerous women who have many of the signs of hypothyroidism by simply having them eliminate their use of birth control pills.

B. Hormone Replacement Therapy

Hormone replacement therapy commonly uses estrogens such as Premarin® or Estrace®. Any orally prescribed estrogen will result in an increase in thyroxine binding globulin (TBG) which will decrease the amount of thyroid hormone that is available for the body to use.[6] This increase in TBG only occurs with the use of oral estrogen preparations. Transdermal (i.e., applied to the skin) therapies do not raise TBG and consequently do not promote a hypothyroid state. I have seen many women with hypothyroid symptoms improve their condition when they stop taking their oral synthetic hormone replacement therapy.

C. Beta- Blockers

Beta-blockers are a class of medications used for a variety of cardiovascular problems including hypertension, coronary artery disease, and congestive heart failure. Examples of beta-blockers include Inderol®, Lopressor®, etc. Beta-blockers inhibit the production of T4 to T3.[7] [8] Beta-blockers are also frequently used for hyperthyroid symptoms.

D. Antimanic Agents

Lithium, in pharmacologic doses, results in a decreased thyroid hormone synthesis and decreases the release of thyroid hormone from the thyroid gland. I have found that many patients on lithium exhibit signs of hypothyroidism, which can be improved by lowering or decreasing the dose of lithium. Physiologic (i.e., small microgram) doses of lithium do not result in a decreased thyroid hormone synthesis.

E. Chemotherapy Agents

I have found most individuals who have received chemotherapy will exhibit signs of hypothyroidism. Many of the agents used in chemotherapy inhibit the production of thyroid hormone. Examples of agents that have been shown to alter thyroid hormone function include Asparaginase, cytokines (interferon, interleukin), 5-fluorouracil (5-FU), 6-mercaptopurine, Mitotane, and Tamoxifen.[9][10]

F. External Radiation

Radiation to the head and neck areas can result in hypothyroidism. Studies have shown hypothyroidism is increased within 3-5 years after external radiotherapy, but can continue to develop for years afterwards. One study found that over 50% of individuals treated with radiation for lymphoma developed hypothyroidism after 20 years.[11] Other studies have shown hypothyroidism rates of 30-40% in individuals treated with radiation.[12][13][14] The addition of chemotherapy with radiation therapy results in a greater incidence of hypothyroidism than occurs with either chemotherapy or radiation alone. My experience has shown that those individuals that have had chemotherapy and radiation therapy in the past have extremely high levels of hypothyroidism.

G. Anemia Drugs

Iron supplements, when taken with thyroid medications result in a decreased gastrointestinal absorption of the thyroid medications.[15] Taking both of these substances together can lead to less thyroid hormone available for the body and thus exacerbate hypothyroid symptoms.

H. Cytokines (Interferon-α and Interleukin-2)

Interferon-α is used for the treatment of hepatitis and for various malignancies. Interferon-α has been associated with hypothyroidism as well as hyperthyroidism. Interleukin-2 is used for the treatment of various malignancies. Individuals treated with Interleukin-2 have a high (32%) percentage of hypothyroidism.[16]

Low Adrenal States

A properly functioning adrenal gland is necessary for the body to convert T4 to T3 as well as for the body to adequately utilize thyroid hormones. In a hypoadrenal state (i.e., low adrenal gland hormonal output), hypothyroid symptoms are very common. Chapter 6 will deal with this concept in more detail.

Growth hormone deficiency

Growth hormone deficiency can lead to a hypothyroid condition. Conversely, hypothyroidism can also cause growth hormone deficiency. Researchers have shown that growth hormone stimulates the conversion of T4 to T3. [17] [18] I have found a synergistic effect using growth hormone along with thyroid hormone, when they are indicated. I have also observed that growth hormone levels will frequently rise after a hypothyroid condition is properly treated. More information about growth hormone can be found in Chapter 7.

Soy

Dietary influences on the functioning of the thyroid gland are important to recognize. Soy has been shown to reduce the conversion of T4 to T3 in animals.[19] A study in humans found that daily soy consumption resulted in symptoms of hypothyroidism (i.e., malaise, constipation, sleepiness) and goiters in 50% of the subjects. These hypothyroid symptoms resolved one month after stopping the soy ingestion.[20] In my experience, many of my patients who ingest non-fermented soy products daily (i.e., soy milk, cheese, tofu, etc.) tend to exhibit more exaggerated signs of hypothyroidism, which will often resolve when soy is limited in the diet. I have not observed the same problems with fermented forms of soy (i.e., miso, tempeh). I recommend limiting--or better yet avoiding-- non-fermented soy products in the diet.

Vitamin and Mineral Imbalances

There are many minerals and vitamins that, when deficient, will cause alterations in the thyroid gland. Although individual nutrients will be discussed, the thyroid gland works optimally when all of the nutrients are properly balanced and available for the body to utilize. In addition, one nutrient, Alpha-Lipoic Acid has been shown to inhibit the conversion of T4 to T3. This section will explore the more common vitamin and mineral deficiencies that can result in abnormal thyroid function.

Iodine

The relationship between thyroid function and adequate iodine levels has been known for over 50 years. In order for the thyroid gland to make thyroid hormone, there must be adequate amounts of iodine present. In fact, T4 thyroid hormone has four iodine molecules attached to it while T3 has three iodine molecules attached to it. When there are inadequate iodine levels in the body, the thyroid gland will be unable to make thyroid hormone and the thyroid gland will be more prone to developing a goiter (i.e., an enlarged thyroid gland). Lack of iodine in the soil and in the food will lead to poor thyroid function.

Many areas of the world have soil that is poor in iodine. These areas have been referred to as 'goiter belt' areas because of the increased prevalence of goiters in people living in these areas. Goiter belts are found in inland areas of countries, such as the Great Lakes basin of the United States. Generally, areas near the ocean have soil that contains adequate amounts of iodine.

Iodized salt has decreased the prevalence of goiters in the goiter belts of the world. However, there is still a great prevalence of iodine deficiency present in the population today. I see it in my practice every day. Chapter 11 will discuss iodine deficiency in more detail.

Selenium

The enzyme that converts T4 to T3, 5'-deiodinase, is dependent on adequate mineral levels, particularly selenium and iodine levels.[21] [22] When selenium levels are inadequate, this enzyme will not function optimally and symptoms of hypothyroidism may develop.

Generally, areas in the goiter belts are not only deficient in iodine; they are also deficient in selenium as well. Eating foods grown in these areas will result in iodine and selenium deficiencies, which can lead to hypothyroid problems. Selenium deficiency is also common in individuals eating a low protein diet.[23] My experience has shown that selenium deficiency is widespread in the population.

Although the addition of iodine to table salt has improved the iodine status in many individuals, it has done nothing to improve the selenium status. I have found significant numbers of patients in my practice who have selenium deficiencies, with resultant hypothyroid symptoms. When these deficiencies are improved, their hypothyroid symptoms often improve.

Jodi, age 37, complained of being fatigued for ten years. "It started after the birth of my child. I had a very difficult pregnancy, and I could never regain my energy level after that. I was told by everybody that it was normal to be tired after having a child, but nothing would help me," she claimed. Jodi had seen numerous doctors and was given medications for depression. "The drugs never helped me. They only made the situation worse," she said. When I saw Jodi, she had many of the signs and symptoms of hypothyroidism, including having cold hands and feet, dry skin, constipation, weight gain and hair loss. Her basal body temperatures averaged 96.6 degrees Fahrenheit (normal temperatures are 97.8-98.2 degrees Fahrenheit—see Chapter 2). A hair and mineral test showed Jodi with very little selenium and iodine stores in her body. Also, her blood tests indicated that Jodi was not adequately converting T4 to its active thyroid hormone T3. When Jodi was given mineral supplements to correct the low levels of selenium and iodine she noticed an immediate improvement. She claimed, "Within 2 weeks of starting the supplements, I started to feel better. My energy level began to improve and my bowels started to work better. Even my husband began to notice that I was feeling better." Jodi was treated with a small amount of Armour® thyroid along with vitamin and mineral supplements. Within six months, her hair and mineral tests showed normal levels of nutrients. Jodi now takes a multiple vitamin mineral product and eats more whole foods that are a rich source of vitamins and minerals. She has continued to maintain good health for the past two years.

Zinc

The serum levels of zinc are positively correlated with the levels of the active thyroid hormone, T3, especially in the aging population.[24] In zinc deficient rats, lowered conversion of T4 to T3 has been observed.[25] My experience has clearly shown a decrease in the conversion of T4 into T3 in zinc deficient individuals.

Vitamin C

Vitamin C is an important antioxidant for the body. Vitamin C can help in the conversion of T4 into T3. When heavy metals, such as cadmium have interfered with the conversion of

T4 into T3, Vitamin C was shown to normalize this conversion.[26] Inadequate Vitamin C levels could cause a decrease in the conversion of T4 into T3.

Vitamins A and E

Vitamins A and E have been shown to be lower in individuals suffering from thyroid abnormalities.[27] Correcting a deficiency in either Vitamin A or Vitamin E will improve thyroid function.

Vitamin B12

When cattle were fed a diet that resulted in a Vitamin B12 deficiency the result was a significant reduction in the conversion of T4 to T3.[28] I believe Vitamin B12 deficiency to be one of the most common nutrient deficiencies in the United States today because of inadequate Vitamin B12 levels in food and a poor absorption of Vitamin B12 associated with aging. Furthermore, B12 levels are lowered in those that take acid-blocking medications. It is impossible to have a properly functioning thyroid gland without adequate Vitamin B12 levels in the body.

Alpha-Lipoic Acid

Alpha-Lipoic Acid is a vitamin-like antioxidant that is produced naturally in the body. It is also found in various food sources including brewer's yeast, liver and potatoes. Alpha-Lipoic Acid is used for various medical conditions including liver disorders (i.e., hepatitis and cirrhosis), diabetes, HIV and heavy metal toxicity. It is also used to help stimulate the detoxification pathways in the body. In some individuals, alpha-lipoic acid can decrease the conversion of T4 to T3. One study found that the use of alpha-lipoic acid decreased the conversion of T4 into T3 by 56%.[29] It has been my experience that the majority of individuals treated with alpha-lipoic acid do not develop thyroid problems. However, I have observed thyroid problems in a subset of patients who do take alpha-lipoic acid. Therefore, thyroid levels must be closely monitored in individuals who take alpha-lipoic acid.

Hemochromatosis

Hemochromatosis is a condition whereby the body absorbs too much iron, resulting in excess iron being deposited in various tissues of the body. Hemochromatosis is a very common condition. In the United States approximately one million people have evidence of hemochromatosis and up to one in every ten people may carry the gene for the disorder. Hemochromatosis has been associated with thyroid disorders and deposition of iron in the thyroid gland has been found in individuals suffering from hemochromatosis.[30]

Cigarette Smoking

In individuals with Hashimoto's thyroiditis, cigarette smoking increases the risk of developing hypothyroidism. A study from Japan showed a 42% increase in hypothyroidism in smokers versus non-smokers.[31] Another study showed those who smoked had higher levels of TSH, indicating smoking worsens hypothyroidism.[32] Cigarette smoking results in the production of thiocyanate in the body which is an inhibitor of iodine uptake.

Thyroid Hormone Resistance

Thyroid hormone resistance is a condition in which the target tissue for thyroid hormone (i.e., the cells of the body) has a reduced responsiveness to thyroid hormone. In other words, thyroid hormone is not able to bind effectively to the cells of the body, resulting in signs of hypothyroidism. Thyroid hormone resistance can occur even with adequate production of thyroid hormone.

Thyroid hormone resistance is analogous to adult onset diabetes (or Type II diabetes). In Type II diabetes, the body produces an adequate amount of insulin. However, the tissues of the body are relatively insensitive to the insulin, resulting in the complications of diabetes. The treatment for adult onset diabetes often revolves around making the tissues less resistant to insulin (i.e. weight loss, exercise) and increasing insulin availability by taking medications or insulin. Similar treatment options are available for thyroid hormone resistance—making the tissues less resistant to thyroid hormone (detoxify the body) and increasing thyroid hormone availability (correct nutrient imbalances or use therapeutic amounts of thyroid hormone).

In 1967, researchers first described the partial resistance of target tissues to the actions of thyroid hormone.[33] It is difficult to measure the true resistance to thyroid hormone, since we have no direct measurement of what the thyroid hormone is actually doing at the cellular level. Thyroid hormone resistance can be inferred through laboratory testing whereby serum T4 and T3 values can vary from just above to several fold above the upper limit of normal, while TSH levels are usually normal.[34] In cases of thyroid hormone resistance, higher than normal doses of thyroid hormone may be required to produce the desired effects on the body.[35] There are also genetic factors that contribute to thyroid hormone resistance.

The treatment of thyroid hormone resistance often includes using the dosages of thyroid hormones that are necessary to override the cellular resistance.[36] Dr. John Lowe has done extensive research on this subject. Dr. Lowe's research indicates that individuals with normal thyroid hormone levels who have fibromyalgia may have thyroid hormone resistance. Case reports published by Dr. Lowe indicate that fibromyalgia patients with normal thyroid blood tests improved their symptoms with the use of thyroid hormone. Dr. Lowe concluded that these individuals probably had a partial resistance to thyroid hormone. Dr. Lowe has confirmed his observations in three placebo-controlled, double- blind crossover studies.[37] [38] [39]

It is interesting to note that in individuals with thyroid hormone resistance, treatment with thyroid hormone can result in blood tests that may indicate a hyperthyroid state (i.e., too much thyroid hormone is being given). However, the people treated did not exhibit any of the signs of hyperthyroidism. It can only be concluded that in these patients, the higher levels of thyroid hormone are necessary to overcome a partial resistance to thyroid hormone at the tissue levels. Remember, in these individuals, the 'normal' ranges in the thyroid tests may not apply.

Perhaps many of the individuals with long-standing fibromyalgia or chronic fatigue syndrome have various degrees of tissue resistance to thyroid hormone. This would explain the improvement in these patients when they are treated with thyroid hormone in the face of normal thyroid blood tests. My experience in treating many patients with fibromyalgia or chronic fatigue syndrome indicates that there are many individuals who do suffer from thyroid hormone resistance. These individuals will see an improvement in their condition with the use of supraphysiologic doses of thyroid hormones, when indicated. Also, they will not exhibit any signs of thyrotoxicosis (i.e., taking too much thyroid hormone). If there are signs of thyrotoxicosis present, the an adjustment of the dosage of thyroid hormone must be undertaken.

The use of thyroid hormone is not the only treatment that needs to be considered when treating patients with thyroid hormone resistance. I have found that proper balancing of the hormonal system with the use of bioidentical, natural hormones (see Chapter 7 for more information) is integral to the healing process. In addition, correcting nutritional imbalances further speeds the healing process. All of the above items help the thyroid gland function better and also help reverse the signs and symptoms of thyroid hormone resistance.

Estelle, 70 years old, had suffered from chronic fatigue for ten years. "I had to retire from my teaching job because I could not function at work. I became so tired that I could not think straight," she said. Estelle had been to numerous doctors. When no laboratory cause of her condition could be elucidated, she was told to see a psychiatrist. "I went to a psychiatrist who put me on various antidepressant medications. None of them helped. In fact, I began to feel worse on the medications," she lamented. Estelle searched from doctor to doctor for help with her condition. When she began to read about the signs of hypothyroidism on the internet, she was sure that she had hypothyroidism. She said, "I kept asking my doctors to check my thyroid hormone levels and they always came back 'within normal limits'. The more I read about thyroid problems, the more I was sure that that was my problem." When I first saw Estelle, she had many of the clinical signs of hypothyroidism including: dry skin, slow reflexes, swelling under her eyes, hair falling out, poor nail growth, a thickened and coated tongue and others. Her basal body temperatures averaged 96.2 degrees Fahrenheit. Estelle's thyroid function tests, however, fell in the normal range. She also had low adrenal hormones (e.g., DHEA, progesterone, testosterone, pregnenolone) and low mineral levels including magnesium, selenium and zinc levels. When she was given a therapeutic trial of Armour Thyroid® hormone, along with correcting the other hormonal and nutritional imbalances, all *of her symptoms began to improve. Furthermore, she has never exhibited any signs of too much thyroid hormone since starting therapy. "Within two weeks, I began to feel better. My head began to clear. I could feel my memory start to return. After a few months, I felt like my normal self again. I haven't felt this good in a long time and I feel like I have been given my life back," she exclaimed.*

Estelle's case is typical of many patients that I see in my practice. The cause of hypothyroidism can be mulitfactorial. In some people, it is caused by a failure of the thyroid gland itself or a failure of the pituitary or the hypothalamus gland. In others, there can be nutritional imbalances at fault. Yet others can be producing enough thyroid hormone, but not be utilizing thyroid hormone due to thyroid hormone resistance. In Estelle's case, using laboratory parameters, her body was producing enough thyroid hormone for her levels to indicate 'normal' thyroid tests. However, her symptomatology and clinical signs indicated that the body was not utilizing the thyroid hormone appropriately. Estelle's case could be explained by the diagnosis of thyroid hormone resistance.

Dr. Lowe's research verifies what I have observed in my practice. He writes, "There is a high incidence of hypothyroidism among fibromyalgia patients. In virtually all cases of hypothyroid fibromyalgia, the symptoms of fibromyalgia are relieved when the patient undergoes metabolic rehabilitation involving three procedures: (1) the use of nutritional supplements, (2) exercise to tolerance, and (3) TSH-suppressive dosages of thyroid hormone.[40]

Thyroid hormone resistance can occur from multiple factors including:

1. Genetic anomalies of thyroid-hormone receptors.
2. Autoimmune, oxidative, or toxic damage to thyroid-hormone receptors.
3. Competitive binding to thyroid-hormone receptors by pollutants, food additives, etc.

All three items will lead to poor utilization of thyroid hormone and fit the criteria for thyroid hormone resistance. In someone with any of these three factors, a therapeutic trial of thyroid hormone may be able to overcome the resistance and reverse many of the signs of hypothyroidism. Furthermore, detoxification of the body can aid in cases of thyroid hormone resistance by helping the receptors of thyroid hormone function more effectively. (See Chapter 9 for more information on detoxification.) I have found the use of detoxification very helpful for helping one overcome thyroid hormone resistance.

Final Thoughts

Physicians have come to rely on laboratory tests as the sole criteria for diagnosing many illnesses. Laboratory tests alone will miss many cases of hypothyroidism, especially in those that suffer from chronic disease. Since there is not one laboratory test that tells us what thyroid hormone is doing at the cellular level— where it has its impact—laboratory tests should <u>not</u> be used as the sole guide to diagnosing and monitoring thyroid disorders. The laboratory tests need to be correlated with other parameters, including the basal body temperatures and the clinical signs and symptoms. This approach will lead to a more thorough evaluation and help begin a more complete treatment program.

This Chapter was written to explain why so many individuals with chronic illness have thyroid problems. Furthermore, I wrote this chapter to help the reader understand why they may have normal thyroid blood tests, yet still be hypothyroid. Many of these people have T4 to T3 conversion problems. In improving this condition, many hypothyroid symptoms will improve.

Also, thyroid hormone resistance is a major reason why so many individuals respond positively to thyroid hormone. Thyroid hormone resistance needs to be recognized and treated appropriately to help individuals overcome hypothyroid symptoms.

If you have many of the signs and symptoms of hypothyroidism (see Table 1 page 34) and have normal thyroid blood tests, do not be discouraged. Perhaps improving your thyroid function can effectively treat your symptoms. This chapter and the remainder of this book can provide you with a roadmap to overcome your illness.

[1] Harrisons Book of Internal Medicine. 14th Edition. 1998.

[2] Blanchard, Kenneth. Quote in <u>Living Well With Hypothyroidism</u> by Mary Shomon. Avon Books, 2000

[3] Olivieri, O, et al. Selenium, zinc and thyroid hormones in healthy subjects: low T3/T4 ratio in the elderly is related to impaired selenium status. Biol. Trace Elem. Res. 1996 Jan;51 (1):31-41

[4] Burroughs, V, et al. Thyroid function in the elderly. Am. J. Med. Sci. 1982 Fan;283(1):8-17

[5] Olivieri, O. IBID.

[6] Utgiger, Robert. Estrogen, thyroxine binding in serum and thyroxine therapy. N.Eng.J. Med. Vol. 344, No. 23. June 7, 2001.

[7] Burger, AG. Effects of pharacologic agents on thyroid hormone metabolism. In: Braverman, LE. Werner and Ingbar's the Thyroid: A Fundamental and Clinical Text. 6th ed. 1991. 477-485

[8] Wiersinga, Wm. Propranolol and thyroid hormone metabolism. Thyroid 1991. Summer; 1(3):273-7

[9] IBID, Braverman.

[10] Kaplan, M. Interactions between drugs and thyroid hormones. Thyroid Today. 1981 (Sept/Oct): 4(5) 1-6

[11] Hanock, S.l, et al. Thyroid disease after treatment of Hodgkin's disease. N. Eng. J. Med. 1991;325:559

[12] Tami, TA, et al. Thyroid dysfunction after radiation therapy in head and neck cancer patients. Am. J. Otolaryngol. 1992;13;357

[13] Chin, D, et al. Thyroid dysfunction as a late effect on survivors of pediatric medulloblastoma/primitive neuroectodermal tumors: a comparison of hyper fractionated versus conventional radiotherapy. Cancer. 1997;80:798

[14] Locatelli, R., et al. Late effects in children after bone marrow transplantation.: a review. Haematologica. 1993;78;319

[15] Orti, E. Thyroid hormone therapy: When to use it, when to avoid it. Drug Therapy. 1994;24(4) 28-35

[16] Schwartzentruber, DJ, et al. Thyroid dysfunction associated with immunotherapy for patients with cancer. Cancer. 1991:115:178

[17] Ho, Ken. Diagnosis and management of adult growth hormone deficiency. Endocrine. April 2000. Vol. 12, No. 2. 189-196.

[18] Moller, Jens, et al. Effects of growth hormone administration on fuel oxidation on thyroid function in normal man. 1992. W.B. Saunders Company

[19] Rumsey, TS, et al. Roasted soybeans and an estrogenic growth promoter affect the thyroid status of beef steers. J. Nutr. 1997; 127:352

[20] Ishizuki, Y. The effects on the thyroid gland of soybeans administered experimentally in healthy subjects. Nippon Naibunpi Gakkai Zasshi. 1991;67:622-629

[21] Berry, MJ et al. Type 1 iodothyronine deiodinase is a selenocysteine-containing enzyme. Nature 1991. Jan 31;349(6308): 438-440

[22] Ruz, M., et al. Single and multiple selenium-zinc-iodine deficiencies affect rat thyroid metabolism and ultrastructure. J. Nutr. 1999. Jan;129(1):174-80

[23] Antioxidant and thyroid hormone status in selenium-deficient phenylketonuric and hyperphenylalaninemic patients. Am. J. Clin. Nutr. 2000. Oct;72(4):976-81

[24] Ravaglia, G., et al. Blood micronutrient and thyroid hormone concentrations in the oldest-old. J. Clin. Endocrinol. Metab. 2000. Jun;85(6):2260-5

[25] Ruz, M., et al. Single and multiple selenium-zinc-iodine deficiencies affect rat thyroid metabolism and ultrastructure. J. Nutr. 1999Jan; 129(1): 174-80

[26] Gupta, P., et al. Role of ascorbic acid in cadmium-induced thyroid dysfunction and lipid peroxidation. J. Apppl. Toxicol. 1998. Sept-Oct;18(5):317-320

[27] Mesaros-Kanjski, E., et al. Endemic goiter and plasmatic levels of vitamins A and E in the school-children on the island of Krk, Croatia. Coll. Antropol. 1999 Dec;23(2):729-36

[28] Stangl, G.I., et al. Cobalt deficiency effects on trace elements, hormones and enzymes involved in energy metabolism of cattle. Int. J. Vitam. Nutr. Res. 1999. Mar;69(2):120-6

[29] Segermann, J., et al. Effect of alpha-lipoic acid on the peripheral conversion of thyroxine to triiodothyronine and on serum lipid-, protein- and glucose levels. Arzneimittelforschung 1991. Dec;41 (12):1294

[30] Edwards, C.Q, et al. Thyroid disease in hemochromatosis. Arch. Intern. Med. 1983;143:1890

[31] Fukata, S, et al. Relationship between cigarette smoking and hypothyroidism in patients with Hashimoto's thyroiditis. J. Endocrin. Inve. 1996:19:607

[32] Muller, B, et al. Impaired action of thyroid hormones associated with smoking in women with hypothyroidism. New. Eng. J. Med. 1995;333:964

[33] Refetoff, S., et al. Familial syndrome combining deaf-mutism, stippled epiphysis, goiter, and abnormally high PBI: possible target organ refractoriness to thyroid hormone. J. Clin. Endocrin. Metab. 1967;27:279

[34] Refetoff, Samuel. IBID. Braverman. P. 1035

[35] Refetoff, Samuel. IBID. Braverman. P. 1029

[36] Lowe, John. IBID. p. 281

[37] Lowe, J.C., et al. Effectiveness and safety of T3 (triiodothyronine) therapy for euthyroid fibromyalgia: a double-blind placebo-controlled response-driven crossover study. Clinical Bulletin of Myofascial Therapy, 2(2/3):31-58, 1997

[38] Lowe, J.C., et al. Triiodothyronine (T3) treatment of euthyroid fibromyalgia: a small replication of a double-blind placebo-controlled crossove study. Clinical Bulletin of Myofascial Therapy, 2(4):71-88. 1997

[39] Lowe, JC., et al. The process of change during T3 treatment for euthyroid fibromyalgia: a double-blind placebo-controlled crossover study. Clin. Bull. Myofascial Ther. 2(2/3):91-124, 1997

[40] Lowe, J.C. IBID. Metabolic Treatment of Fibromyalgia. McDowell. 2000. p. 283.

Chapter 4

Thyroid Replacement Options

Chapter 4

Thyroid Replacement Options

Angela, age 25, was taking Armour® Thyroid (1/2 grain/day) for Hashimoto's disease and hypothyroidism. Although she felt better on the thyroid medication, she still had complaints of aches and pains as well as fatigue. Upon changing her thyroid medication to Nature-Throid™ (1/2 grain/day), all of her symptoms improved within one week. "I knew I did not feel 100% on the Armour® thyroid, but I was better. It took seven days before the Nature-Throid™ kicked in. I woke up one day and all my aching and fatigue was gone. I couldn't believe it," she said.

Armour® Thyroid and Nature-Throid™ are both desiccated porcine thyroid medications. The only difference between the two medications is the filler content. Armour® Thyroid has cornstarch in it while Nature-Throid™ does not. I have found many individuals with thyroid disorders sensitive to the inactive ingredients (i.e., fillers) in the medications. Each person has a unique biochemical profile that requires an individualized treatment program. If you are not responding to one thyroid medication, don't be discouraged. Sometimes just changing the brand of medication can make all the difference between feeling good and feeling ill. This chapter will explore the various thyroid medications available and show you the differences between the medications.

There are many choices when it comes to choosing a thyroid hormone to treat hypothyroidism or autoimmune thyroid disorders. Most conventional physicians rely solely on Levothyroxine (T4) preparations (e.g., Synthroid® or Levothroid®). However, my experience has shown that when treating a patient with a thyroid disorder the best result is to look at each patient as a unique biochemical individual. There is no "one size fits all" treatment for thyroid disorders. I believe each patient requires his/her individualized therapy specific for their own needs. So many people are suffering from poor outcomes to thyroid treatment because the regimen prescribed to them does not meet their unique needs.

Over 15 years of practicing holistic medicine has proven to me, beyond a doubt, that thyroid replacement therapy can (and should) be individualized to fit a patient's needs. How is it done? I use the techniques that I was taught in medical school. I start by a taking a history. Next, I perform a physical exam and then, I order laboratory tests. Finally, I look at the whole picture before formulating a treatment plan. When the treatment plan includes the use of thyroid hormone, there are many choices available. This chapter will review these choices and help educate the reader on which therapies are available and why some therapies may be more appropriate for certain individuals.

Remember, the best results with treating thyroid disorders are always achieved by working with a health care practitioner who is knowledgeable in the many treatment options available. This chapter will be organized into the different thyroid hormone preparations that are available to treat thyroid disorders.

Levothyroxine (T4) Preparations

The most widely used and well-known thyroid hormone replacement medications are known as T4 preparations. The "4" in T4 refers to the number of iodine molecules present in each thyroid molecule. Recall from Chapter 2, the thyroid gland releases T4 which is converted into the more active T3 thyroid hormone (see Figure 1, page 36). Table 1 gives examples of many of the T4 preparations currently available.

Table 1: T4 Thyroid Hormone Preparations
Levothroid®
Levoxyl®
Synthroid®
Unithroid®

Each T4 thyroid preparation is supposed to be standardized to contain the stated amount of hormone. However, each manufacturer adds different inactive ingredients that may cause problems if there are allergies or adverse reactions to these ingredients. For example, some of the inactive ingredients in Synthroid® are shown in Table 2.

Table 2: Inactive Ingredients of Synthroid®
Cornstarch
Dyes including aluminum lake
Lactose

There are many people who have dairy allergies. In fact, it is the most common food allergy that I diagnose. Those who have a dairy allergy should not consume lactose and lactose-containing products.   Unithroid® also contains lactose. Levothroid® would be a better T4 choice for those with dairy allergies as it does not contain lactose.

As mentioned in Chapter 2, there are many people who cannot convert some, most, or all of T4 into T3. In these cases, T4 preparations may not be the optimum choice for thyroid hormone replacement. In my experience, many patients will have a better response to thyroid medications that contain the more active thyroid hormone T3.

Levothyroxine (T4) and Triiodothyronine (T3) Combination Preparations

Hormone therapies containing both T4 and T3 thyroid hormone have been around for many years. Table 3 lists some of the T4 and T3 combination hormones.

Table 3: T4 and T3 Combination Thyroid Hormone Preparations

Armour® Thyroid
Nature-Throid™
Westhroid™
Thyrolar®

Perhaps the best known combination thyroid hormone is Armour® Thyroid. Armour® Thyroid is a porcine (pig) derived thyroid hormone. Each grain of Armour® Thyroid hormone contains 38μg of T4 and 9μg of T3. As previously mentioned in

Chapter 2, Armour® thyroid®, being glandular derived, also contains other active ingredients including: calcitonin, selenium and the thyroid hormones T2 and T1. Both Nature-Throid™ and Westhroid™ contain the same amounts of thyroid hormone as Armour® thyroid as well as the same other active ingredients listed above. Nature-Throid™ and Westhroid™ are identical agents.

Armour® Thyroid, Westhroid™, and Nature-Throid™ are very similar items. They are all derived from porcine thyroid glands. The biggest difference between these agents is that Armour® Thyroid contains dextrose made from cornstarch. This may allow Armour® Thyroid to be absorbed sublingually. Neither Westhroid™ nor Nature-Throid™ contain any corn ingredients. Those with an allergy to corn products might be better served by Westhroid™ or Nature-Throid™.

Although Armour® Thyroid, Westhroid™ and Nature-Throid™ are very similar items; there can be a large difference in the individual's response to each hormone. My experience has shown that those individuals who are hypothyroid can usually be treated with either of the three hormones and have a successful result. However, those with a corn allergy should avoid Armour® Thyroid. Furthermore, those with an autoimmune thyroid disease (e.g., Hashimoto's) may experience better results with a corn-free version such as Nature-Throid™ or Westhroid™. If you are not having success with one version of desiccated thyroid hormone, I would suggest trying another version.

Thyrolar® is a synthetic thyroid preparation that contains both T4 and T3. The ratio of T4 to T3 is 4:1. For those opposed to a porcine product, Thyrolar® is an option. Thyrolar® contains cornstarch and lactose as inactive ingredients. Those with a corn and/or dairy allergy should not take this product.

Lena, Angela's mother (recall Angela from case history at the beginning of this chapter), was taking Armour® Thyroid for hypothyroidism. "I did not see a difference taking it. I took it because you told me to take it," she told me. Her blood tests improved from the Armour® Thyroid, but many of her symptoms including poor growing and cracking nails, lowered energy and brain fog, did not improve. When she was changed to Nature-Throid™, she noticed an immediate improvement. "Now, I can tell when I take thyroid medication. Before, I couldn't tell a thing. I feel so much better on Nature-Throid™. The best thing is my brain feels so much better as I am so much clearer in my thinking," she said. Lena's case is not uncommon. Finding the best thyroid medication for the individual provides the best outcome.

Triiodothyronine (T3) Thyroid Preparations

Cytomel® is the most widely used form of T3. There is also a generic T3 known as Liothyronine sodium. Studies have shown the addition of small amounts of T3 to T4 (e.g., Synthroid® or Levothroid®) therapies improved symptoms of depression, mood, and cognitive performance.[1][2] However, Cytomel® may not be the best choice for T3 therapy. One of the problems with Cytomel® is that it only comes in two doses: 5µg and 25µg. Many patients may need a different amount of T3 to effectively treat their condition. Also, Cytomel® contains sucrose and talc as inactive ingredients. I have seen many patients allergic to talc. The sucrose is used to make Cytomel® a rapidly absorbed substance. Cytomel® is rapidly absorbed, almost 95% absorbed, in four hours.[3] This rapid absorption can cause a "roller-coaster" effect with Cytomel®, which many patients do not like. This "roller coaster" effect can present in patients as palpitations or anxiety followed by fatigue. I find compounded, slow release T3 preparations much more effective and easier to tolerate than Cytomel®.

Compounded Thyroid Medications

Compounding pharmacies have been preparing compounded thyroid hormones for over 100 years. Compounding pharmacies can make various doses of pure T4 and T3 thyroid hormones, without additives and fillers. The benefit of using a compounding pharmacist is that each patient can receive a unique dose that provides an individualized ratio specific for their condition.

One of the main benefits of using a compounding pharmacist is the use of slow-release T3 hormone. My experience has clearly shown that slow-release T3 hormone is much more effective and easier to titrate as compared to rapidly-absorbed T3 hormone such as Cytomel®. Furthermore, I have witnessed far fewer side effects with compounded, long-acting T3 thyroid hormone as compared to Cytomel®. Finally, a compounding pharmacist can work with patients who have unique allergy concerns and formulate products that are hypoallergenic. I work closely with compounding pharmacists on a daily basis.

Final Thoughts

As shown in this chapter, there are many different thyroid hormones available. Each patient needs an individualized treatment plan that takes into account their unique biochemical individuality. No one thyroid preparation or single dose is the best for everyone. Many times it takes a trial and error period to find the optimum dose and medication. If you are not receiving the best results, I suggest trying a different medication, or consider altering the dosage.

For those patients who are highly allergic or very sensitive to odors and chemicals, working with a compounding pharmacist may provide the best result. A skilled compounding pharmacist can be a great addition to your health care team. To find a compounding pharmacist, see Appendix B.

---

[1] Cooke, RG. T3 augmentation of antidepressant treatment in T4-replaced thyroid patients. J. Clin. Psych. 1992. Jan;53(1):16-8.

[2] Bunevicius, R. Effects of thyroxine as compared with thyroxine plus triiodothyronine in patients with hypothyroidism. N. Eng. J. Med. 1999. Feb. 11;340(6):424-9

[3] From: http://www.fda.gov/cder/foi/label/2002/10379s47lbl.pdf. Accessed 11.21.07

Chapter 5

Hyperthyroidism and Autoimmune Disorders

Hyperthyroidism and Autoimmune Thyroid Problems

The thyroid gland is one of the most important hormone producing glands in our body. The thyroid gland produces thyroid hormone that influences the metabolism of every single cell in the body. In a hypothyroid state, there is too little thyroid hormone. In a hyperthyroid state, there is too much thyroid hormone produced. Symptoms of hyperthyroidism include nervousness, sweating, palpitations, nerve tingling, fatigue, heat intolerance, hyperactivity, eye disorders and an increased appetite.

Hyperthyroidism can be caused by a variety of illnesses. Examples of illnesses that can cause a hyperthyroid condition are listed in Table 1. Many of the conditions listed in Table 1 are considered autoimmune disorders, such as Graves' disease and Hashimoto's disease.

Table 1: Examples of Disorders that can lead to Hyperthyroidism

Chronic thyroiditis with transient thyrotoxicosis
Graves' disease
Hashimoto's disease
Hyperfunctioning adenoma
Subacute thyroiditis
Toxic multinodular goiter

Autoimmune Disorders

The immune system is our body's defense mechanism against infection. When a foreign invader (i.e., bacteria, virus, parasite, etc.) attacks the body, the immune system goes into high gear in order to fight the infection. The immune system responds to these foreign invaders by producing substances known as antibodies, which fight the foreign organisms. These antibodies bind to the foreign substance and effectively neutralize the organism. This is one of our body's main defenses against infection.

An autoimmune disorder refers to a condition whereby the immune system malfunctions and begins to produce antibodies against its own tissue. These same antibodies that are supposed to protect against infection now begin to attack the body's own tissue.

Graves' disease and Hashimoto's disease are examples of autoimmune disorders of the thyroid gland. In Hashimoto's disease and Graves' disease, the body produces antibodies that attack the thyroid gland. These antibodies are known as antithyroid antibodies and antimicrosomal antibodies. These antibodies bind to cells on the thyroid gland, which causes inflammation, and often destruction of the thyroid gland. As the thyroid gland becomes more inflamed, it releases excess thyroid hormone. This excess thyroid hormone often causes the signs and symptoms of hyperthyroidism. Table 2 lists some of the signs and symptoms of hyperthyroidism. Autoimmune thyroid problems often lead to hyperthyroidism initially and can be followed by hypothyroidism later in the course of the illness.

Table 2: Signs and Symptoms of Hyperthyroidism

Fatigue	Nervousness
Goiter	Palpitations
Heat Intolerance	Sweating
Hyperactivity	Tremor
Hypertension	Weakness
Menstrual Disturbance	Weight Loss

There are many disorders of the thyroid gland that can cause hyperthyroidism. Examples of thyroid problems that can cause hyperthyroidism are shown in Table 1 (page 116). This Chapter will focus on the two most common forms of autoimmune disorders that can lead to hyperthyroidism: Hashimoto's disease and Graves' disease.

How Prevalent Are Autoimmune Disorders?

Autoimmune disorders are among the leading cause of death among American women under age 65.[1] Women are diagnosed with autoimmune disorders much more frequently than men. Approximately 5% of women in the United States have an autoimmune disorder today. This Chapter will focus on the autoimmune illnesses of the thyroid gland; however, there are many other autoimmune illnesses in the body. Examples of these are shown in Table 3.

Table 3: Autoimmune Illnesses	
Crohn's	Polymyositis
Graves'	Psoriatic Arthritis
Hashimoto's	Reiter's
Juvenile Arthritis	Rheumatoid Arthritis
Juvenile Diabetes	Scleroderma
Lupus	Sjogren's
Multiple Sclerosis	Ulcerative Colitis
Polymyalgia Rheumatica	Vasculitis

How Does One Get an Autoimmune Disorder?

In conventional medicine, there is no consensus as to why someone becomes ill with an autoimmune disorder or what actually causes an autoimmune disorder. Consequently, the treatment for autoimmune disorders in conventional medicine has not been very effective. If you don't understand the underlying cause of an illness, then how can an effective treatment modality be developed?

In conventional medicine, the approach to treating autoimmune disorders primarily relies on treating the symptoms of the disorder. Toxic medications such as steroids and chemotherapeutic agents such as methotrexate are often prescribed. These items primarily block inflammation in the body. However, inflammation is not the cause of the illness, it is the consequence of the illness.

As I described in my book ***Overcoming Arthritis,*** the infectious etiology of various autoimmune disorders has been around for over 100 years. Pioneering physicians such as Dr. Thomas Brown described their success in treating many patients who suffered from various autoimmune disorders with small doses of antibiotics. Dr. Brown's 50 years of research showed that many patients suffering from autoimmune illnesses were infected with a particular bacterium called mycoplasma. By using small doses of antibiotics to treat the mycoplasma infection, Dr. Brown succeeded in treating many difficult autoimmune illnesses.

Table 4 shows many of the autoimmune illnesses that may have an infectious etiology. In my experience, I have found underlying infections in many of these illnesses. In many cases the infectious agent may be part of or the underlying **cause** of the autoimmune disorder. By treating this underlying infection, many times the symptoms of the autoimmune illness will significantly improve or resolve.

Table 4: Diseases That May Have An Underlying Infectious Etiology

Chronic Fatigue Syndrome	Polymyalgia Rheumatica
Crohn's	Polymyositis
Fibromyalgia	Psoriatic Arthritis
Gulf War Syndrome	Reiter's
Graves' Disease	Rheumatoid Arthritis
Hashimoto's	Scleroderma
Juvenile Arthritis	Sjogrens
Lupus	Ulcerative Colitis
Multiple Sclerosis	Vasculitis

Table 5 lists some of the infectious agents that have been shown to cause various autoimmune disorders, including autoimmune thyroid disorders, arthritic disorders, fibromyalgia, chronic fatigue syndrome and others.

Table 5: Infectious Agents which can Cause Arthritic Disorders

Borrelia burgdorferi	Mycobacterium Tuberculosis
Brucella	Mycoplasma
Candida	Neisseria
Chlamydia	Parvovirus B19
Coxiella	Staphylococcus Aureus
Fungi	Streptococcus
Hepatitis B	Treponema pallidum
HIV	Viruses

Why Test for a Mycoplasma Infection?

My clinical experience has shown that, in many cases, the underlying cause of an autoimmune illness can be an infection. Although there are many different infectious agents implicated in autoimmune disorders, the bacterium mycoplasma stands out as one of the most prevalent bacteria.

Mycoplasma was first associated with the arthritic disorders in the 1800's. After isolating the mycoplasma bacterium from the infected joints of rheumatoid arthritic patients, Dr.

Brown began successfully treating patients with small amounts of antibiotics directed against the mycoplasma bacterium. Dr. Brown also found this bacterium in a wide range of other arthritis-related disorders including Lupus, Scleroderma and others.

When I started to check my patients who suffered with a variety of autoimmune disorders for the mycoplasma bacterium, I found that surprisingly high percentages (approximately 75%) of these patients showed laboratory evidence of an active infection. Most of these patients improved with antibiotic and nutritional therapy directed against the mycoplasma bacterium. Researchers have been reporting that from 50% to 70% of individuals suffering from fibromyalgia and chronic fatigue syndrome are found to have mycoplasma infections.[23] I have found very similar percentages of mycoplasma infections in patients with autoimmune thyroid conditions such as Graves' disease and Hashimoto's disease.

Iodine Deficiency and Autoimmune Disorders

In my book, *Iodine: Why You Need It, Why You Can't Live Without It, 3rd Edition*, I describe how iodine deficiency predisposes the thyroid gland for undergoing oxidative damage. This oxidative damage is analogous to a small fire burning in the thyroid gland. The body's defense against this oxidative damage (or fire burning) is to produce antibodies against its own thyroid tissue—anti-TPO or anti-TBG. The cornerstone of this treatment is to reverse the oxidative damage with antioxidants and correct iodine deficiency. The supplements most helpful for achieving this include:

Vitamins B2 (500mg/day) and B3 (300mg/day)

Magnesium (200-400mg/day)

Vitamin C (3-5,000mg/day)

Iodine (dosage varies)

A more detailed explanation of the therapeutic use of iodine in treating autoimmune thyroid disorders can be found in ***Iodine: Why You Need It, Why You Can't Live Without It, 3rd Edition***. The best result with any treatment modality is to work with a health care professional knowledgeable in the use of these nutrients.

Graves' Disease

Graves' disease is named after the researcher who first described the illness. Graves' disease is an autoimmune illness, which is characterized by an enlarged thyroid gland and the production of thyroid antibodies. This often causes a hyperthyroid condition.

Like most thyroid problems, Graves' disease is more common in women. It is reported to occur in 5 out of 10,000 people, but its incidence has been increasing. It is especially prevalent in women between the ages of 20 to 40 years old and in women who have just given birth. Table 6 shows other autoimmune illnesses that predispose one to Graves' illness.

Table 6: Autoimmune Illnesses Associated with Graves ' disease
Addison's disease Lupus Pernicious anemia Rheumatoid arthritis Type 1 diabetes Vitiligo

The symptoms of Graves' disease are varied. Many of the symptoms are similar to the symptoms of hyperthyroidism (see Table 2 page 117). In addition to the symptoms of hyperthyroidism, people suffering from Graves' often have:

- Protruding Eyes

- Goiter (swelling of the thyroid)

- Abnormal nerve sensations (tingling, buzzing in extremities, etc.)

Physical exam signs for Graves' disease often show an elevated heart rate and an enlargement of the thyroid gland. The blood tests for Graves' disease often show a depressed TSH and elevated T3 and T4 levels. Often a radioactive iodine uptake test is done which will show an increased uptake by the thyroid gland.

Cheryl a 46-year-old mother of two was diagnosed with Graves' disease 2 years ago. Cheryl initially had many of the symptoms of hyperthyroidism. "I was extremely nervous and jittery. I couldn't sit still and I could not sleep at night. Also, I had constant tingling in my arms and legs," she said. Cheryl was treated with radioactive iodine, which did little to help her symptoms. "The radioactive iodine did take away some of the nervousness, but all of the other symptoms continued. I was so miserable, the doctors decided to remove my thyroid, which did not help much." When Cheryl initially saw me, she was miserable. She was taking a drug (PTU) to block the hyperthyroid effects, but she was having side effects from the drug. I diagnosed Cheryl with a Mycoplasma infection and started treating her with Minocycline, an antibiotic that treats Mycoplasma infections. Cheryl immediately noticed an improvement. She said, "The Minocycline was the first thing that I have taken that started to make a difference. All of my symptoms began to calm down after the Minocycline was started." Cheryl was treated with vitamins, minerals and herbs designed to boost the functioning of her immune system. After one year of taking antibiotics at low doses, Cheryl tested negative for the mycoplasma bacterium. Cheryl has continued with her nutritional regimen and feels much better. "I know I am not 100% better, but I am so much better I am thrilled. I can now ride a bike without getting exhausted and I can do so much more with my sons," she happily exclaimed.

Hashimoto's Disease

Hashimoto's disease is named after Hakaru Hashimoto, the 20th century Japanese surgeon who first recognized the disease. Hashimoto's disease is an autoimmune disorder in which the body produces a specialized type of white blood cell (lymphocyte) which attacks the thyroid gland. This results in an inflammatory response to the thyroid gland.

The symptoms of Hashimoto's disease are varied. A swollen thyroid gland, otherwise known as a goiter, is very common with Hashimoto's. The thyroid will enlarge in size as the disease process impairs its function. The most common complaint people have is fullness in the throat area. Initially, patients may feel signs of too much thyroid hormone—hyperthyroidism. Symptoms include racing of the heart, nervousness, etc. This is due to an inflammation of the thyroid gland, causing the gland to release much of its stored thyroid hormone. After a period of time, and after the thyroid gland essentially 'burns' itself out, the hyperthyroid symptoms will give way to hypothyroid symptoms, such as fatigue, coldness, etc.

It is common for blood tests to show elevated levels of thyroid antibodies in those who suffer from Hashimoto's. These antibodies include:

- Antithyroid Antibodies
- Antimicrosomal Antibodies

Hashimoto's disease can affect people of all ages. It has its most common incidence among women in their thirties and forties. Up to two percent of the population may suffer from Hashimoto's.

Hashimoto's disease, like Graves' disease, is also associated with other autoimmune illnesses. Table 7 shows which autoimmune illnesses are associated with Hashimoto's.[4]

Table 7: Autoimmune Illnesses Associated with Hashimoto's

Adrenal insufficiency
Chronic active hepatitis
Diabetes
Graves'
Lupus
Rheumatoid arthritis
Sjögren's Syndrome

Mary, age 36, developed thyroid problems after the birth of her second child, two years ago. "After the birth of my son, I could not recover. I could not lose weight and I could not get my energy level back. I kept going to the doctor and he kept telling me I was tired because I had a baby to take care of. But I knew something else was wrong," she said. Mary was diagnosed with Hashimoto's disease six months after the birth of her child. By that time, Mary had developed a goiter (swelling of the thyroid gland) and she had antibody levels in her thyroid blood tests (antithyroid antibodies and antimicrosomal antibodies). Mary was told her thyroid blood tests were normal, and that she needed no treatment at that time. She said, "My doctor told me I had to wait until the blood tests showed signs of hypothyroidism before I could begin taking thyroid medication. I told him that I already had many signs of thyroid problems including weight gain, tiredness, coldness and others. I had also checked my basal temperature and it was reading 96.6 degrees Fahrenheit (normal 97.8-98.2 degrees Fahrenheit). My doctor kept telling me to wait and I kept saying 'Wait for what? I am already feeling sick'." When I saw Mary, she had many of the clinical signs of hypothyroidism including puffiness under the eyes, poor eyebrow growth, a thickened, coated tongue, dry skin and slow reflexes. I placed Mary on Armour® thyroid and she immediately felt better. "It was like a cloud was lifted off of my head. I was able to think more clearly and I began to lose weight. Most of all, I was able to take care of my children again," she said. Mary has continued on a small dose of Armour® thyroid (45mg per day) and continues to feel much better.

Lisa, age 32, mother of two, had been an athlete her whole life. She played soccer in college and had always been a very athletic and active person. Lisa had been diagnosed with an autoimmune blood clotting disorder—antiphospholipid syndrome 10 years ago. She was told by her physician to take an aspirin a day and that she had to be careful if she became pregnant. "I never felt the antiphospholipid syndrome had limited my life in any way," she claimed. About two years ago, Lisa began to feel ill. She said, "I started to feel tired all of the time. I would go to bed tired and wake up even more tired. Some mornings it took everything I had to make it down the short hall to my children's rooms. I also experienced severe joint pains—to the point that my husband would have to help me get my pajamas on and help me get into bed. This is not an easy thing for an extremely strong willed, independent woman to admit. Sometimes the joint pain would leave one joint, only to travel to others. It was relentless." Lisa also had other symptoms. "My body would go through drastic temperature changes. I would be cold during the day and have frequent hot flashes at night. I knew something was not right." Lisa consulted her doctor who drew blood tests and told her that her TSH level was too high, indicating a hypothyroid condition. Also, there were antibody levels in her blood stream, which could indicate an autoimmune condition such as Lupus.

She was treated with Synthroid®, which improved her blood tests, but did little for her symptoms. "I kept telling the doctor that I felt no better on the Synthroid. He told me that my symptoms could not be due to hypothyroidism because my thyroid blood tests (TSH and T4 levels) were normal. When I saw Lisa, she had many classical signs of hypothyroidism including poor eyebrow growth, puffiness of the face and under the eyes, slow reflexes, dry skin and poor nail growth. Laboratory tests revealed a normal T4 level and a low T3 level, indicating a poor conversion of T4 into the more active T3. When I changed Lisa's thyroid medication to Armour Thyroid® her T3 levels improved and she noticed an immediate improvement in her symptoms. "My energy began to improve and my muscle aches and pains went away in under two weeks. Also, I lost 10 pounds. I knew that I was on the mend." Lisa was also found to have antibody levels to mycoplasma bacterium, and was treated with low dose antibiotics. Since beginning treatment, Lisa remarked that she felt over 90% better with her symptoms. She recently wrote me a note stating, *"I spent four hours playing in the snow with my children the other day. It was priceless. There was no way I could have done that when I was ill."*

Lisa's case is typical of many patients I see in my office. I have found that many autoimmune disorders may be secondary to a thyroid disorder and that once the thyroid disorder is appropriately diagnosed and treated, the signs and symptoms of the autoimmune disorder improve.

Treatment of Autoimmune Thyroid Problems

The treatment of autoimmune thyroid problems can be complex, especially when hyperthyroid symptoms are prevalent. Oftentimes there are different degrees of severity of symptoms in someone suffering from autoimmune thyroid problems. As mentioned earlier, the important component of the treatment plan is to search for an underlying cause of the illness and supplement the body with basic nutritional therapies. This can involve dietary changes, medication and nutritional supplements.

Gluten Sensitivity

In addition to iodine, I have also seen an association between sensitivity to gluten-containing products and autoimmune thyroid problems. Gluten is the major protein found in many grains, including wheat, rye, barley and others. Gluten intolerance is also known as celiac disease.

Researchers have found that a significant number of patients with autoimmune thyroid disease also have celiac disease. A recent study showed (through blood testing) that people with autoimmune thyroid disease had a 1,300% increase in celiac disease compared to individuals without autoimmune thyroid problems. The authors concluded that patients that have autoimmune thyroid problems should be screened for celiac disease in order to "eliminate symptoms and limit the risk of developing other autoimmune disorders."[5]

Studies have also shown an improvement in thyroid illnesses when a gluten free diet is followed. Researchers have documented improvement in hypothyroidism and have been able to show a decreased need for thyroid medication when the proper diet is followed (i.e., a gluten free diet).[6]

Not everyone that has an autoimmune thyroid problem has celiac disease. Research has shown that from 3%-5% of those with autoimmune thyroid problems may have celiac disease. My experience has shown that a trial of a gluten free diet is warranted for anyone suffering from any autoimmune problem. I have seen positive responses in nearly all my patients who become gluten-free. More information about a gluten-free diet can be found in ***The Guide to a Gluten-Free Diet.***

Following the dietary recommendations in Chapter 8 is also very important for those with autoimmune thyroid disorders. It is vitally important to eat a healthy diet and to avoid items that disrupt the normal functioning of the immune system, such as refined sugar and trans fatty acids. This is discussed in more detail in Chapter 8.

The Problems with Aspartame

In addition to the dietary recommendations mentioned above, anyone suffering from an autoimmune thyroid problem (as well as any autoimmune disorder) must avoid all products that contain aspartame. Aspartame may cause or contribute to autoimmune thyroid problems. In the body, aspartame is metabolized into the toxic substance formaldehyde. It is the toxicity of aspartame to the liver and other organs of the body that may exacerbate symptoms in autoimmune illnesses such as Hashimoto's disease or Graves' disease.

Dr. Hal Roberts, an expert on medical problems associated with aspartame ingestion notes that "Physicians should interrogate patients with recent Graves' disease about aspartame consumption. If [aspartame is] being used, these individuals ought to be observed for a possible spontaneous remission after stopping aspartame before definitive interventions (radioiodine treatment or surgery) are recommended."[7] I could not agree more with Dr. Roberts. For more information on aspartame I refer to the reader to Chapter 8 and to Dr. Roberts' book, Aspartame Disease, an Ignored Epidemic.

Sucralose (Splenda®)

Sucralose is chlorinated table sugar. Chlorine is part of the halide family. Iodine is also found in the halide family. Ingesting too much chlorine-containing products can cause the body to excrete iodine. My clinical experience has shown that the ingestion of sucralose can cause/worsen iodine deficiency problems and also cause/worsen thyroid problems. The heating of chlorine-containing products can produce more toxic chemicals such as dioxin-like products. There are better choices for a sweetener such as xylitol. For more information on which sweeteners to use, I refer the reader to ***The Guide to Health Eating.***

Medication

Although I believe it is better to use natural means to help the body overcome illness, there is a place for the use of drug therapies in autoimmune thyroid illnesses.

When someone is suffering from hyperthyroid symptoms (i.e., nervousness, jitteriness, tremors, etc.) it is important to quickly address these symptoms. Hyperthyroid symptoms can be very disconcerting to the patient. Oftentimes, dietary changes and nutritional supplements will not work quickly enough for the individual. In these cases, drug therapy can be appropriate.

Drugs to relieve the symptoms of hyperthyroidism work very quickly. Though these agents do not treat the underlying cause of the illness, they do work to relieve many of the severe symptoms of hyperthyroidism. Beta-blockers (e.g., Inderol®) can treat the symptoms of rapid heart rate, sweating and anxiety. Antithyroid medications such as Propylthiouracil help with more severe cases. Finally, if medications are unable to control serious hyperthyroid symptoms, surgery may be necessary to alleviate these symptoms.

Small doses of hydrocortisone, an adrenal hormone, can help control the inflammation that is associated with hyperthyroidism. This is especially helpful in the inflammation around the eyes that Graves' disease patients often experience. Physiologic doses of hydrocortisone also help support a hypoadrenal condition that often coexists with autoimmune thyroid illnesses. In individuals that suffer from autoimmune conditions, it is important to diagnose and treat a hypoadrenal condition. Chapter 7 will discuss the hypoadrenal condition.

Radioactive iodine is frequently used by conventional physicians in the treatment of hyperthyroid symptoms. Radioactive iodine is effective at killing the thyroid gland; however, it does have adverse effects. The radioactive iodine not only binds to the thyroid gland, it also binds to areas of the body where iodine is used, such as the ovaries in women. There is some concern that radioactive iodine may cause cancer. Therefore, I feel radioactive iodine should be the last resort for those suffering from hyperthyroid symptoms.

Nutritional Supplements

Taking the correct nutritional supplements can be effective in treating the symptoms of hyperthyroidism. Conversely, taking the wrong supplements can worsen the symptoms.

An interesting substance, Paraaminobenzoic Acid (PABA-- a member of the B Vitamin family) is effective in relieving many of the hyperthyroid symptoms. I have found PABA to be effective in improving the symptoms of hyperthyroidism in approximately 50% of those that suffer from autoimmune thyroid disorders (as well as other autoimmune disorders).

Thymus extract is another nutritional supplement that can be extremely helpful to those suffering from autoimmune thyroid disorders. I have also found Vitamin A helpful to lessen the symptoms from autoimmune thyroid problems.

Selenium can be a useful nutrient for individuals with autoimmune thyroid disorders. Selenium has been shown to slow the progression of autoimmune thyroid disorders. In these disorders, anti-thyroid antibody levels are produced which damage the thyroid gland. Selenium supplementation has been shown to lower these antibody levels.[8] Selenium is deficient in our diet due to low levels of selenium in the soil. I have been measuring selenium levels in the hair and blood of patients for years and I have frequently found low levels in patients suffering from autoimmune disorders. I recommend supplementing with 200-400mcg of selenium per day for those who have autoimmune thyroid disorders.

Other helpful nutrients for autoimmune thyroid disorders include:

1. Vitamin C: 3,000-5,000mg per day.
2. Vitamin B12 (hydroxyl or methyl cobalamine): injected—1,000-5,000mcg per day for 30 days

3. Magnesium (chelated): 200-400mg per day

4. Vitamin B6: 50mg per day

5. Cats Claw: 600-900mg per day

6. L-Carnitine 1-2gm/day

Final Thoughts

Treating autoimmune thyroid disorders is challenging. Treatments must be individualized. Sometimes it takes trial and error to find the best treatment program for the individual. Treating the underlying cause(s) of the illness (e.g., an infection), if it can be found, is the best course. By implementing dietary and nutritional support, most individuals with autoimmune thyroid disorders can significantly improve their condition with the holistic approach outlined in this chapter.

[1] American Journal of Public Health. September, 2000;90:1463-1466

[2] Vojdani, Aristo, et al. "Multiplex PCR for the detection of M. fermentans, M. Hominis, and M. Penetrans in patients with chronic fatigue syndrome, Fibromyalgia, Rheumatoid Arthritis, and Gulf War Syndrome." Journal of Chronic Fatigue Syndrome, Vol. 5., No ¾ 1999.

[3] Nicolson, Garth, et al. Mycoplasma Infections in Chronic Illnesses: Fibromyalgia and Chronic Fatigue Syndromes, Gulf War Illness, HIV-AIDS and Rheumatoid Arthritis. Medical Sentinel. Volume 4, No. 5, September/October 1999.

[4] Harrison's Textbook of Internal Medicine. 14th Edition, 1998

[5] Berti, I., et al. Usefulness of screening program for celiac disease in autoimmune thyroiditis. Dig. Dis. Sci. 2000. Feb;45(2):403-406

[6] Valentino, R., et al. Prevalence of celiac disease in patients with thyroid autoimmunity. Hormone Res. 1999;51 (3):124-7

[7] Roberts, H. Aspartame Disease, An Ignored Epidemic. Sunshine Sentinel Press, 2001. p. 432

[8] Rowen, Robert. From Second Opinion Newsletter. Vol. XII, No. 1. p. 7

Chapter 6

Fibromyalgia and Chronic Fatigue Syndrome

Fibromyalgia and Chronic Fatigue Syndrome

This Chapter will explore two common illnesses, chronic fatigue syndrome and fibromyalgia and their relationship to hypothyroidism.

Fibromyalgia is a chronic disorder, characterized by poor sleep, muscle pain, stiffness and tender trigger points on the body. Although fibromyalgia was not recognized by the American Medical Association as a distinct syndrome until 1987, the symptoms of fibromyalgia—muscle pain, difficulty sleeping, tender trigger points—have been reported for hundreds of years.

The criteria for the diagnosis of fibromyalgia as stated in the American College of Rheumatology (ACR) are shown below.

ACR Definition of Fibromyalgia Syndrome

1. A history of widespread pain for at least three months. Pain is considered widespread when all of the following are present: pain in the left side of the body, the right side of the body, below the waist and above the waist. In addition, there should be axial pain (cervical spine or anterior chest or thoracic spine or low back pain).
2. Pain in trigger points on the neck, back, hips, arms and legs.

Chronic fatigue syndrome is characterized by severe fatigue that is unrelieved by rest. Chronic fatigue syndrome has no known cause in conventional medicine. There are certain criteria that must be met to properly diagnose someone with chronic fatigue syndrome. The Center for Disease Control's criteria for the diagnosis of chronic fatigue syndrome is shown on the next page.

It is my belief that fibromyalgia and chronic fatigue syndrome are inter-related syndromes that often have a common underlying factor: hypothyroidism. This Chapter will explore the relationship between hypothyroidism, fibromyalgia and chronic fatigue syndrome in more detail.

Revised CDC Criteria for Chronic Fatigue Syndrome

A case of chronic fatigue syndrome is defined by the presence of the following:

1. Clinically evaluated, unexplained, persistent or relapsing fatigue that is of new or definite onset; is not the result of ongoing exertion; is not alleviated by rest; and results in substantial reduction of previous levels of occupational, educational, social or personal activities.
2. Four or more of the following symptoms that persist or recur during six or more consecutive months of illness and that do not predate the fatigue:
   a. Self-reported impairment in short-term memory or concentration
   b. Sore throat
   c. Tender cervical or axillary nodes
   d. Muscle pain
   e. Multijoint pain without redness or swelling
   f. Headaches of a new pattern or severity
   g. Unrefreshing sleep
   h. Postexertional malaise lasting > 24 hours

Fibromyalgia

The incidence of fibromyalgia is growing at an alarming rate. It is estimated that approximately 3 to 6% of the U.S. population is affected with fibromyalgia.[1][2] Fibromyalgia primarily

145

affects women, especially women in their childbearing ages. There is no consensus in conventional medicine about the cause of fibromyalgia. Some of the reported causes are shown in Table 1.

Table 1: Possible Causes of Fibromyalgia
Allergic Disorder Autoimmune Disorder Bowel Dysbiosis Emotional Distress Infections (viral, bacterial, parasitic) Nutrient Deficiencies Toxicity (heavy metals, chemicals, pesticides, etc.) Trauma (physical or psychological)

The conventional approach to treating fibromyalgia involves primarily treating the symptoms of the disorder, such as poor sleep and muscle aches. This is done with sedatives to improve sleep, anti-inflammatory medications to help relieve the aches and pains, and antidepressants to help elevate the mood. Occasionally, physical therapy or exercise is recommended to improve muscle fitness. The problem with these treatments is that none of the above conventional therapies are designed to treat an underlying cause of the illness; they only treat the symptoms of the illness. The end result of these types of treatments is that the illness will often continue to progress.

There have been no long-term studies validating the effectiveness of using drug therapies to treat fibromyalgia. That is not to say that drug therapies do not have their place; they do. Drugs may be necessary to help improve poor sleep patterns or to temporarily relieve pain in fibromyalgia patients. However, for the best outcome to be achieved, the underlying cause of the illness must be identified and treated.

The Relationship between Hypothyroidism and Fibromyalgia

The symptoms of fibromyalgia and hypothyroidism are very closely related. In fact, compared to the general population, a number of studies have reported that a significant percentage of individuals with fibromyalgia also have hypothyroidism.

One study found that over 63% of individuals diagnosed with fibromyalgia had laboratory signs of hypothyroidism.[3] The same researchers completed a second study to look at this relationship and found that over 50% of fibromyalgia patients had laboratory signs of hypothyroidism. The authors of this study point out that, "Contrary to anecdotal reports, hypothyroidism is extraordinarily common among fibromyalgia patients."[4]

As discussed in Chapter 2, relying solely on conventional laboratory tests will miss many individuals who are actually suffering from hypothyroidism. This also holds true for fibromyalgia individuals. My experience has shown that over 60% of fibromyalgia patients have hypothyroidism.

Which Comes First: Hypothyroidism or Fibromyalgia?

If, as I propose, over 80% of individuals with fibromyalgia have hypothyroidism, the question becomes 'Which comes first; hypothyroidism or fibromyalgia?' This is a difficult question to answer.

Muscle aches and pains and fatigue are the cardinal signs of fibromyalgia. Perhaps the muscle aches and pains and fatigue that are present in fibromyalgia patients are caused by hypothyroidism.

The association between hypothyroidism and muscle achiness was reported in the medical literature nearly 100 years ago. Fatigue associated with hypothyroidism was also reported over 100 years ago. In a lecture to the International Surgical Congress in 1914, it was reported that a patient who suffered from fatigue as well as stiff, hard and painful muscles improved with thyroid treatment. The doctor described how the general pain and stiffness disappeared steadily with the use of thyroid hormone. Furthermore, when the patient ceased treatment with thyroid hormone, the problems gradually returned. The physician concluded that the pain was "simply a manifestation of defective thyroid secretion."[5] This case study showed the benefit of using thyroid hormone to effectively treat fibromyalgia.

Dr. John Lowe, a noted researcher on the connection between fibromyalgia and hypothyroidism, recently reported that the incidence of hypothyroidism in individuals suffering from fibromyalgia is extremely high. In looking solely at blood tests, he found that over 50% of individuals with fibromyalgia tested positive for hypothyroidism.[6] If you take into account the physical exam signs, the history and the basal body temperatures, the prevalence of hypothyroidism in individuals suffering from fibromyalgia would be significantly higher. As previously mentioned, I have found that the actual prevalence of hypothyroidism in fibromyalgia patients is well over 80%.

If my hypothesis-- that the prevalence of hypothyroidism in fibromyalgia patients is present in many individuals-- is correct, then why would conventional medicine not recognize this trend? The answer to this question goes back to the information discussed in Chapter 2 on the failure of laboratory tests to properly diagnose hypothyroidism. Primarily relying on the TSH test to diagnose hypothyroidism will miss a significant proportion of individuals suffering from hypothyroidism.

The diagnosis of fibromyalgia became much more prevalent after conventional medicine began to rely on the TSH test to diagnose thyroid problems. Before this reliance on the blood tests occurred, the diagnosis of hypothyroidism was primarily a clinical diagnosis. In other words, the physician was treating the patient and not the laboratory test. By relying on the blood tests, many cases of hypothyroidism began to be missed. As time progressed those individuals with untreated hypothyroidism began to develop signs and symptoms of fibromyalgia.

My experience has shown that individuals with fibromyalgia can exhibit all of the signs of hypothyroidism, yet have normal blood tests. Eventually, as the situation worsens, the blood tests (i.e., TSH test) will finally 'catch up' to the symptoms and reflect a hypothyroid condition. This process can take years. During this time, if the hypothyroidism is not properly recognized and treated, the symptoms of fibromyalgia (i.e., muscle aches and pains, and fatigue) will continue to worsen.

So, what comes first, hypothyroidism or fibromyalgia? Since the symptoms of fibromyalgia are the same symptoms as hypothyroidism, it is logical to assume that hypothyroidism precedes the diagnosis of fibromyalgia. As mentioned above, the symptoms of fibromyalgia-- muscle aches and pains, and fatigue-- have been described in the medical literature for almost 100 years, primarily as a hypothyroid condition. It is my belief that, in many individuals, fibromyalgia develops as a chronic disorder after a long period of untreated hypothyroidism.

As discussed in Chapter 2, the blood tests will miss many individuals with hypothyroidism. It is these individuals who have a hypothyroid condition that, over time, will develop a chronic illness like fibromyalgia. The treatment of hypothyroidism, if instituted early in the course of the illness, can often reverse all the signs of muscle aches and pains, and fatigue (i.e., fibromyalgia).

David Derry, M.D., Ph.D., a thyroid expert and researcher, feels that the reliance on the thyroid blood tests, particularly the TSH test, has resulted in the huge rise of fibromyalgia (and chronic fatigue syndrome). Dr. Derry describes how, a few years after the medical profession began to rely on the TSH test to diagnose hypothyroidism (instead of evaluating the clinical signs and symptoms), the diagnosis of fibromyalgia and chronic fatigue syndrome began to appear. "Chronic fatigue and fibromyalgia were nonexistent {diseases} before 1980. So where did these two new diseases come from? The symptoms and signs of fibromyalgia and chronic fatigue were described in the literature in the 1930's as one way that low thyroid could be expressed. Treated early, it was easily fixed with thyroid in adequate doses. But even then, the clinicians had noticed that if a patient had low thyroid for too long, then it became more difficult to treat all the signs and symptoms regardless of what they were."[7] Dr. Derry feels the reliance on the TSH test in conventional medicine "needs to be scrapped and medical students taught again how to clinically recognize low thyroid conditions."[8]

Although there can be a multitude of causes for fibromyalgia, my experience has shown that the vast majority of patients suffering from fibromyalgia have a hypothyroid condition. It is my opinion that the diagnosis of fibromyalgia is often caused by a long-standing hypothyroid state. People with fibromyalgia need to be properly diagnosed and treated for hypothyroidism, and the lab tests should not be the sole basis for this diagnosis.

Rosa, a 45-year-old mother of two, complained of muscle aches. "I always have achiness in my muscles. After I do any type of activity, all the muscles of my body become irritated. They hurt so much that I have difficulty brushing my hair," she said. Rosa had not felt well since the birth of her second child 10 years ago. "I know something happened to me after the birth of my son. I just couldn't recover. My energy level evaporated and my muscle strength decreased. I went to doctor after doctor and no one could give me an answer. They kept telling me I needed to see a psychiatrist," she lamented. Rosa also complained of being cold all the time, including having extremely cold hands and feet. She was also constipated and was losing her hair. All of these symptoms are classic signs of hypothyroidism. "I kept asking my doctors to check my thyroid hormone levels, but the hormone levels always tested normal in the blood tests. Every time I read about hypothyroidism, I felt like I was reading about myself," she commented. When I evaluated Rosa, she had many clinical signs and symptoms of hypothyroidism. Furthermore, her basal body temperature (see Chapter 2) averaged 96.5 degrees Fahrenheit (normal 97.8-98.2 degrees Fahrenheit). Rosa's thyroid blood tests were in the lower part of the normal range. When Rosa was therapeutically treated with a small amount of Armour Thyroid® hormone, her symptoms dramatically improved. "In less than two weeks, I began to wake up and clear the fog I was in. My muscle aches began to improve and I was no longer freezing cold all the time. Most importantly, I began to get my life back and be able to be a proper mother to my children," she happily said.

The Treatment of Fibromyalgia

As mentioned before, there are many possible causes of fibromyalgia (see Table 1 page 146). To properly treat an illness, one must understand its underlying cause(s). As I described earlier, I have found that hypothyroidism is a primary cause of fibromyalgia in at least 80% of patients with fibromyalgia.

In my experience, it is impossible for one to recover from fibromyalgia if the thyroid gland is not functioning properly. The symptoms of fibromyalgia (i.e., muscle achiness and fatigue) are very similar to the symptoms of hypothyroidism. It must be kept in mind that an adequate amount of thyroid hormone is necessary, both for the muscles of the body to function appropriately and for the production of adequate amounts of energy. In assessing fibromyalgia patients, I believe it is absolutely necessary to first evaluate the functioning of the thyroid gland. If there is a hypothyroid condition present, this must be treated before all else. For more information on treating hypothyroidism, please see Chapter 2.

It is well known that the immune system will not function effectively in a hypothyroid state. Perhaps this is why so many fibromyalgia patients have signs of an infectious etiology; their thyroid gland is not working appropriately. Another possible cause of fibromyalgia is poisoning by heavy metals such as mercury, which can negatively impact the thyroid gland. Nutrient deficiencies can also lead to a poorly functioning thyroid gland. The cause(s) of fibromyalgia can be varied. The best results are achieved with a comprehensive evaluation looking at many varied factors.

Chronic Fatigue and Immune Dysfunction Syndrome (CFIDS)

CFIDS affects approximately one million Americans.[9] Although CFIDS can affect all people of any age, race or socioeconomic status, it primarily affects women, at a rate of 3:1 over men.

In conventional medicine, there is no consensus on what causes CFIDS, or on the proper treatment regimen. As previously mentioned, it is important to ask the question, "If you don't know the cause of the illness, then how can you fashion an effective treatment?"

Many research studies report multiple triggers that cause the illness. Table 2 illustrates some of these triggers. Notice the same triggers that may cause fibromyalgia, can also cause CFIDS.

Table 2: Triggers for CFIDS

Allergic Disorder
Autoimmune Disorder
Bowel Dysbiosis
Emotional Distress
Infections (viral, bacterial, parasitic)
Nutrient Deficiencies
Trauma (physical or psychological)
Toxicity (heavy metals, chemicals, etc.)

Conventional Treatment Options for CFIDS

The conventional therapy for CFIDS includes using different medications to treat its symptoms. Generally this involves the use of drugs for depression and anxiety. Anti-inflammatory agents are also used occasionally to relieve muscle aches and pains. In addition, when sleep is difficult for the patient, sleeping medications may be prescribed.

The problem with relying solely on drug therapies is that the drug therapies only treat the symptoms of the illness; they do not address the underlying cause(s). Drug therapies may be necessary in the short-term to help relieve the symptoms of chronic fatigue syndrome, but they are not effective for overcoming CFIDS. In fact, I have found that long-term drug use can often make CFIDS more difficult to overcome.

I believe that instead of using drug therapies to treat the symptoms of CFIDS, we should try to identify and treat the underlying cause(s) of the illness. It has been my experience that hypothyroidism is a primary underlying cause of CFIDS in a majority of cases.

The Relationship between Hypothyroidism and CFIDS

The relationship between CFIDS and hypothyroidism has been known for many years. In fact, the symptoms of CFIDS were described over 100 years ago in the medical literature as hypothyroid symptoms. Fatigue, the primary complaint in CFIDS, is present in almost all individuals with hypothyroidism.

Fatigue can be a complaint of numerous medical conditions, including anemia, cancer, infections etc. It is not always related to hypothyroidism. However, in the case of CFIDS, I have found that a large percentage of my patients have been hypothyroid. Furthermore, most of these patients will experience a significant improvement in their symptoms when the hypothyroid condition is appropriately diagnosed and treated.

The difficulty with treating CFIDS patients for hypothyroidism is that the results of their blood tests are often in the normal range; although they may have many clinical signs and symptoms of hypothyroidism. Researchers have reported relief of symptoms when patients with chronic fatigue were treated with thyroid hormone.[10]

Dr. John Lowe, a researcher in the connection between thyroid problems and chronic illness, believes that "...the most common cause of fatigue is inadequate thyroid hormone regulation of cell function."[11] Dr. Broda Barnes (Chapter 2) wrote that fatigue is "a common problem of the hypothyroid and has long been known to be."[12]

There are multiple reasons why hypothyroidism can cause fatigue. In the hypothyroid state, the basal metabolic rate of the body slows down. This slowing of the basal metabolic rate will result in a fatigue state. Also, in the hypothyroid individual, the heart will not pump the blood as efficiently as it should. This will decrease oxygen flow to the tissues of the body; ultimately resulting in fatigue.

It has been my experience that the majority of CFIDS patients have low basal body temperatures (see Chapter 2). A low basal body temperature is one indication that the thyroid gland may be malfunctioning. It is also an indication that the basal metabolic rate has slowed, which is very common in the hypothyroid individual. My experience has shown that over 80% of individuals with CFIDS have low basal body temperatures and have many of the clinical signs and symptoms of hypothyroidism.

Treatment of CFIDS

In order to effectively treat CFIDS, one must address the underlying cause(s) of the disorder. It has been my experience that hypothyroidism is a major underlying cause of many cases of CFIDS. A hypothyroid individual will have a low metabolic rate and, consequently, have complaints of fatigue. In addition, the low thyroid hormone levels will predispose the individual to muscle aches and pains, which are common in CFIDS. Furthermore, the immune system will not be functioning properly in the hypothyroid individual, which can further result in an increased risk of infection.

Caitlin, a 47-year-old professor, developed CFIDS eight years ago after a bad case of the flu. "I was fine one day, then ill with the flu the next day. I thought it was a simple flu, but I never came back. I became so tired that I could not even work," she said. Caitlin took a leave of absence from teaching in order to recover. "I slept away about six months of my life," she claimed. Caitlin went from doctor to doctor but found no relief in any drug therapies. "They put me on antidepressants, but they did not help. I was told to exercise, but I couldn't because I was too tired." Caitlin was able to return to work, but severely restricted her activity. "I used to exercise and enjoy being very active. Now, I feel like I have become old. I have just enough energy to go to work and that is it. I have no more left." When I saw Caitlin, she had many of the signs and symptoms of hypothyroidism including dry skin, cold extremities, irregular periods, fatigue, weight gain and poor eyebrow and hair growth on her body. She also had a low basal body temperature of 96.6 degrees Fahrenheit (normal 97.8-98.2 degrees Fahrenheit). Caitlin's thyroid blood tests were on the low range of normal. When she was given a therapeutic trial of Armour Thyroid® hormone, she noticed an immediate improvement in her energy level. She said, "I felt like a light switch was being turned on in my body. I could think better and I wasn't so tired all the time." Caitlin was also found to be suffering from a mycoplasma bacteria infection. When she was treated for the mycoplasma bacteria, she noticed further improvements. Caitlin was further treated with vitamins and minerals to correct nutritional imbalances and given diet therapy. Today, nearly three years after starting treatment, Caitlin feels 80% improved. "I can now exercise and I am much more productive at work. I get comments from my friends and family about how much better I look. I feel like I have my life back," she said.

The holistic approach to treating CFIDS is to treat the underlying cause(s) of the illness. This involves treating hormonal imbalances, particularly hypothyroid conditions. If the thyroid gland is not properly functioning, these individuals will not be able to overcome this devastating illness. In addition, nutrient deficiencies, other hormonal imbalances, and infections must be addressed. These items will be covered next.

Why do so Many Individuals with Fibromyalgia and Chronic Fatigue Syndrome have Hypothyroidism?

As previously stated, I believe that 40% of the population is suffering from hypothyroidism. A large percentage of these hypothyroid individuals are untreated. It is this population that is at greatest risk for developing chronic disorders such as fibromyalgia and CFIDS.

At times of added stress on the body, the weakest part of the body will be affected first. Some hypothyroid individuals have a tendency to develop fibromyalgia, while others may develop CFIDS. Although the same condition (i.e., hypothyroidism) can predispose one to differing illnesses (i.e., fibromyalgia or CFIDS), the different presentation has to do, in part, with the genetic makeup of the individual as well as environmental influences.

Nutrient deficiencies can also set the stage for problems with the thyroid gland. For example, mineral deficiencies, such as selenium or iodine, can lead to a hypothyroid state. Chapter 8 describes the many nutrient deficiencies that can lead to hypothyroidism. I believe that nutrient deficiencies are rampant in the United States due to poor farming techniques and the overuse of fertilizers on our crops. The thyroid gland cannot appropriately manufacture and release its hormone without adequate amounts of minerals in the diet.

Fluoride has been added to our water supply to help prevent cavities in the teeth. As a mineral, fluoride is similar to iodine. In fact, the ingestion of fluoride has been shown to decrease the ingestion of iodine. The thyroid gland has the highest concentration of iodine in the body and uses iodine to manufacture the active thyroid hormones. In medicine, fluoride was once used to slow down an overactive thyroid gland. Perhaps one reason there are so many hypothyroid individuals is because of the process of adding fluoride to the water supply.

Exposures to heavy metals also cause thyroid problems. Mercury, a toxic heavy metal, has been shown in numerous studies to cause thyroid dysfunction. Mercury toxicity is rampant in the United States due, in large part, due to the use of amalgam fillings by dentists. Amalgam fillings contain approximately 50% mercury. In my practice, I have diagnosed a significant number of patients with mercury toxicity. When this toxic load is reduced through a detoxification plan many systems in the body improve, including the thyroid and other endocrine glands.

Finally, many drugs used in conventional medicine can inhibit thyroid function. These drugs include: estrogens, beta-blockers, asthma medications, and others.

How Do You Treat Someone With Fibromyalgia or CFIDS?

The treatment of fibromyalgia or chronic fatigue syndrome can be complex. Often, there are multiple problems occurring at the same time (e.g., nutrient deficiencies, hormonal imbalances, etc.). In order to best treat these difficult conditions, I have found it is absolutely necessary to search for an underlying cause and to correct any hormonal imbalance that is present. This underlying cause can take many different forms including heavy metal toxicity, viral or bacterial infections, nutrient deficiencies, and others. Oftentimes, a hormonal imbalance, particularly a thyroid hormonal imbalance, can be found to be the underlying cause of the illness.

The first step to an adequate treatment program is to perform a thorough evaluation. A thorough evaluation should include gathering a history and performing a physical exam. In addition, blood tests to evaluate nutrient function, immune system function, and hormonal levels should also be performed. To further assess the nutrient and heavy metal status, I have found a hair analysis to be extremely helpful. Combining all of the above modalities together will ensure a complete evaluation of complex chronic illnesses such as fibromyalgia or CFIDS.

Because the thyroid gland affects every cell in the body and is vitally important for proper functioning of the immune system, ensuring a properly functioning thyroid gland should be a primary step in the treatment of fibromyalgia and CFIDS.

It is very common for an individual with CFIDS or fibromyalgia to be told that their thyroid gland is functioning normally. However, as previously stated, relying solely on thyroid blood tests is not the correct way to fully evaluate the thyroid gland. The thyroid gland can be better evaluated by correlating the physical exam signs and symptoms, the basal body temperatures and the blood tests.

As a physician, I believe it is important to realize that I am treating a patient not a blood test. In my experience, many patients with fibromyalgia and CFIDS can significantly improve or overcome their illness when a thyroid disorder is properly diagnosed and treated.

In evaluating the hormonal system in fibromyalgia or CFIDS, the thyroid gland is not the only gland that should be evaluated. These patients often have multiple hormonal systems out of balance, including the adrenals, sex glands (ovaries in women and testes in men), pituitary, hypothalamic and others. The entire endocrine system needs to be appropriately evaluated and balanced with natural hormones to achieve the best results. Please see Chapter 7 or *The Miracle of Natural Hormones, 3rd Edition* for more information on other hormones.

[1] From National Institutes of Health and Department of Health and Human Services and the National Fibromyalgia Association

[2] Weir, P. The Incidence of Fibromyalgia and Its Associated Comorbidities: A Population Based Retrospective Cohort Study Based on International Classification of Diseases, 9th Revision Codes. June, 2006 issue of the Journal of Clinical Rheumatology

[3] Lowe, John. Thyroid status of 38 fibromyalgia patients: implications for the etiology of fibromyalgia. Clinical Bulletin of Myofascial Therapy, 2(1) 47-64. 1997

[4] Lowe, John, et al. Thyroid Status of Fibromyalgia patients. Myofascial Therapy, 3(1): 47-53. 1998

[5] Hertoghe, Eugene, M.D. 1914. Thyroid Deficiency Lecture presented to the International Surgical Congress

[6] Lowe, John. Thyroid status of fibromyalgia patients. Myofascial Therapy, 3(1): 47-53, 1998

[7] Interview with Dr. David Derry. In About .Com, by Mary Shomon. July, 2000

[8] Derry, David. "TSH has no clinical correlation." Letter to British Medical Journal. October 17, 1999

[9] Richman, J., et al. A community based study of chronic fatigue syndrome. Arch. Int. Med. 1999; 159(18):2129

[10] Lindstedt, Goran. Thyroid dysfunction and chronic fatigue. Letter. Lancet. Vol. 358. July 14, 2001

[11] Lowe, John. The Metabolic Treatment of Fibromyalgia. Mcdowell. 2000. p. 608

[12] Barnes, Broda. Hypothyroidism, The Unsuspected Illness. Harper and Row. 1976. p. 52

Chapter 7

Adrenal and Gonadal Hormones and their Relationship to the Thyroid

Adrenal and Gonadal Hormones and their Relationship to the Thyroid

Although this book focuses on recognizing and treating thyroid problems, it is important to look at all of the hormonal glands because they are all closely related. If there is a need to use a hormone for any condition, I recommend using natural, bioidentical hormones. I have found a synergistic effect that is readily apparent when small (i.e., physiologic) doses of natural, bioidentical hormones are employed to balance the endocrine system.

This Chapter will review the adrenal and pituitary hormones that I have found to have a synergistic effect with thyroid hormone in treating chronic illness as well as improving the functioning of the body. The hormones covered in this Chapter include:

1. DHEA

2. Hydrocortisone
3. Testosterone
4. Natural Progesterone
5. Natural Estrogens
6. Human Growth Hormone
7. Pregnenolone

For more information on the use of natural hormones, I refer the reader to my book, ***The Miracle of Natural Hormones, 3rd Edition.***

When I began to recognize the magnitude of thyroid problems in my patients, I found good results in improving my patients' chronic illnesses by balancing their thyroid levels. However, I then started looking at the hormonal system in its entirety and I found that other hormonal glands (e.g., adrenals, ovaries, pituitary and testicles) were also imbalanced.

I have found using natural hormones to be a safe and effective therapeutic regimen to correct these imbalances. A natural hormone is generally made from a plant product and has the same chemical structure of the hormones produced in our bodies. Because the hormone has the same chemical structure of our own hormones, it is much less likely to cause adverse effects, as compared to commonly used synthetic hormones, such as

Provera® and Premarin®. Figure 1 below illustrates the difference between a natural and a synthetic hormone. Most synthetic

Figure 1: A Comparison of a Natural Hormone (Natural Progesterone) and a Synthetic Hormone (Provera®)

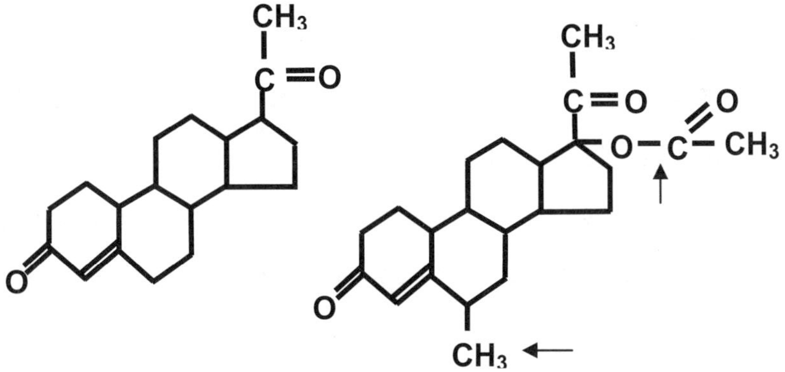

Progesterone

Provera®

The difference between the natural hormone, progesterone, and the synthetic version, Provera® is illustrated in this diagram. The arrows in the Provera® illustration point out the additional side chains added to progesterone. These added chains make Provera® a foreign substance in the body, leading to an increased risk of adverse effects.

hormones can be considered 'foreign substances' to the body, since the body does not recognize the chemical structure of the substance.

It makes common sense to argue that natural, bioidentical hormones should be the first line of treatment for any hormonal therapy because the body more readily accepts them. Furthermore, using natural hormones in combination is much more effective than using these hormones individually.

There is a close relationship between the thyroid gland and the other glands of the body, particularly the adrenal glands, the sex glands (ovaries and testes), and the hypothalamus and the pituitary gland. Using combinations of natural hormone therapies to restore the endocrine balance can significantly improve the condition of many individuals who are suffering from chronic illnesses, including thyroid disorders. In addition, this approach can help reverse many of the signs of aging.

The Relationship between the Thyroid Gland and the Adrenal Glands

It is impossible to achieve optimum health without a properly functioning hormonal system. In order for the hormonal system to operate properly, all of the endocrine glands (e.g., thyroid, adrenals, ovaries, testes and pituitary) must be functioning at their optimal levels. Although each of the endocrine glands are vital in their own right, this Chapter will focus on the relationship between the thyroid gland and the adrenal glands.

The adrenal glands lie at the upper pole of both kidneys and they produce hormones that allow an individual to adapt to changes in the environment. The adrenal glands are sometimes referred to as the 'fight or flight' glands. The adrenal hormones are responsible for the 'rush' necessary to run away from or to begin a fight. These hormones are involved in the different responses to anger, fright and fear. They are responsible for the increased heart rate, increased blood pressure and mobilization of sugar from the liver to the blood stream, which can prepare us for the 'fight or flight'.[1]

The adrenal glands produce a variety of hormones including; DHEA, hydrocortisone, estrogen, testosterone, progesterone and pregnenolone. All of these hormones interact with thyroid hormone in the body. An inadequate production of adrenal hormones can result in a poor conversion of the inactive thyroid hormone, T4, into the more active thyroid hormone T3 (See Chapter 3 for more information on T4 conversion problems).

When thyroid hormone is prescribed for a hypothyroid state, the metabolism of the body is increased. This increased metabolism will, in turn, stimulate the adrenal glands to secrete its hormones including hydrocortisone. Hydrocortisone is necessary to mobilize glucose out of the cells in order to supply energy to the all of the cells of the body. If the adrenal glands are unable to increase their production of adrenal hormones (i.e., a hypoadrenal state), increasing the metabolism of the body with thyroid hormone can overload the poorly functioning adrenal glands and precipitate a failure of the adrenal glands. The consequences of this failure can be severe, as adrenal failure is incompatible with life. In other words, the adrenal glands must be able to keep up with the increased metabolic needs of the body.

In order to check the adrenal hormonal status, a 24-hour urine test can be ordered to check the adrenal hormone output. If the levels of adrenal hormones are sub-optimal, strong consideration should be made for supplementing with physiologic (i.e., small) doses of adrenal hormones. In these cases, thyroid hormone should not be prescribed until the adrenal glands are properly supported.

Elaine, age 37, suffered from fibromyalgia for 10 years. She became ill after a viral infection. "I remember it clearly. I thought I had the flu, but I never felt the same afterwards. I became increasingly fatigued and developed pain all over my body. I went to many doctors before I could get a diagnosis of fibromyalgia. I feel as if my whole immune system fell apart after I had the flu," she said. Elaine had a low basal body temperature—96,3 degrees Fahrenheit (normal 97.8-98.2 degrees Fahrenheit). She also had many other signs of hypothyroidism including hair loss, cold hands and feet, constipation, dry skin, weight gain and puffiness under the eyes. She claimed, "I feel like a different person than I was 10 years ago. I have turned into an old woman. I can't exercise because it hurts too much. I can barely go to work every day because I am so tired." Another doctor tried her on thyroid hormone, but all of her symptoms worsened. Elaine also had extremely low blood pressure— 90/60—which is a cardinal sign of hypoadrenalism. "I often find myself dizzy when I stand up after lying down. I have to hold on to the wall for a minute or I feel like I will fall down," she claimed. Elaine suffered from a hypoadrenal condition called 'orthostatic hypotension' that is a common problem in individuals suffering from fibromyalgia and chronic fatigue syndrome. Furthermore, Elaine had low thyroid blood tests. Her 24-hour urine test showed low 17 hydroxy-steroids (2.5mg/24 hours, normal 3-10mg/24 hours) and 17 keto-steroids (4mg/24hours), indicating hypoadrenalism. Elaine was treated with two adrenal hormones—DHEA and Hydrocortisone for one week. After one week, she started taking Armour® thyroid. Within four weeks, most of Elaine's symptoms were significantly improved. "Within a couple of days after starting the hormones, I knew I was on the right track. I began to feel the illness lift off of me. After two months, I could exercise again. I didn't realize how sick I really was until I started to feel so much better," she said.

Elaine's case is very common. When there is concomitant hypothyroidism with hypoadrenalism, the correct way to reverse the condition is to supplement with physiologic doses of adrenal hormones first, then add in the thyroid hormones later. In other words, correct a hypoadrenal condition before utilizing thyroid hormone replacement. In using thyroid hormones first, there is the potential to exacerbate the low adrenal output. The remainder of this chapter will explore each of the adrenal hormones and their properties.

DHEA

DHEA is a steroid hormone produced in the adrenal glands. DHEA is an acronym for Dehydroepiandrosterone. DHEA levels, like the other hormone levels in the body, peak at a young age and fade throughout life. (See Figure 2 page 178) I have consistently observed low DHEA levels in elderly patients as well as most individuals suffering from a chronic disease such as a thyroid disorder, fibromyalgia, chronic fatigue syndrome, Lupus, Crohn's, ulcerative colitis, rheumatoid arthritis, cancer or multiple sclerosis. DHEA has been shown to have a protective effect against cardiovascular disease, obesity, hypercholesterol, cancer, diabetes, Lupus and other autoimmune illnesses.[2][3][4][5]

DHEA and Hypothyroidism

Twenty years of research has pointed to the relationship between low DHEA levels and hypothyroidism.[6][7] As explained earlier, hypothyroidism and hypoadrenalism occur commonly together. It is not surprising that there is a relationship between low DHEA levels and hypothyroidism. In any thyroid disorder, my experience has shown that there is a synergistic effect when using physiologic amounts of DHEA along with thyroid hormone. In other words, it is better to use a combination of thyroid hormone with DHEA rather than using either hormone individually.

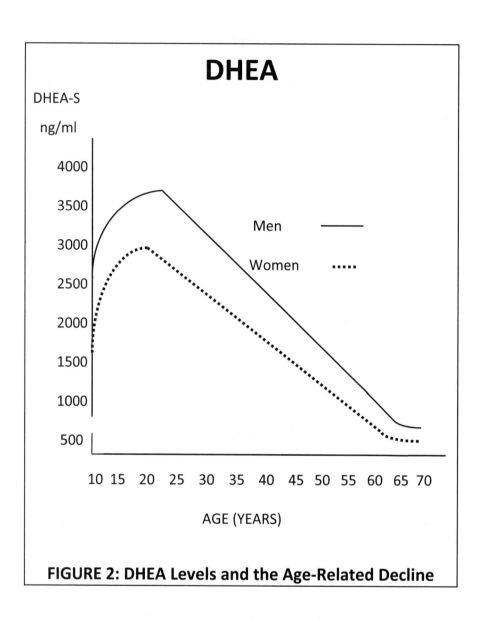

FIGURE 2: DHEA Levels and the Age-Related Decline

However, using too much DHEA can reverse this synergistic effect with thyroid hormone. Only physiologic doses of DHEA should be used in combination with thyroid hormone. I have found that most patients can be successfully managed on very low doses of DHEA in combination with thyroid hormones. Women generally need from 2-5mg per day of DHEA; men generally need from 5-10mg per day.

In prolonged stressful states, the adrenal glands may under-function and produce sub-optimal levels of their hormones, including DHEA. The adrenal hormones DHEA and testosterone are known as anabolic (i.e., tissue building) hormones. When the body has been injured, adequate amounts of the anabolic hormones are necessary for the tissue to heal. William Jeffries, a former professor of endocrinology at Case Western Reserve University, has published numerous articles and books describing how the body will have a difficult time healing when the levels of the adrenal hormones are inadequate. He recommends using small amounts of the adrenal hormones to aid the body in healing.[8] My clinical experience validates Dr. Jeffries' findings.

In my practice, I have found that close to 100% of patients with autoimmune disorders (including fibromyalgia, CFIDS, Crohn's, ulcerative colitis, Lupus, multiple sclerosis and rheumatoid arthritis) have significantly depressed DHEA levels. In addition, most of these patients show clinical improvement in their condition upon using physiologic (i.e., small) replacement doses of DHEA. Researchers have reported similar positive results when using DHEA to treat chronic conditions.[9]

DHEA Dosage and Recommendations

DHEA levels should be investigated in all people who have a chronic illness. However, the reader should be aware of differences in the reported normal ranges of different laboratories. I have found that the adequate levels of DHEA necessary to overcome illness are from 2,000-3,000ng/dl for men and from 1,500-2,500ng/dl for women. All levels in this book are measured as the sulfate form of DHEA-- DHEA-S. These levels closely approximate the peak levels of DHEA seen in Figure 2. In treating thyroid disorders and other chronic illnesses, I have often found it necessary to raise DHEA levels to approximate the peak levels mentioned above.

DHEA levels should be measured before supplementation with DHEA and should be checked at routine intervals during the treatment regimen in order to optimize the dose. I recommend pharmaceutical grade DHEA made by a compounding pharmacist. I have often found that DHEA sold over-the-counter at health food stores is not reliable (approximately 80% of the time). DHEA should be taken on an empty stomach for better absorption. DHEA works best in small amounts (men: 5-10mg/day and women: 2-5mg/day) and has synergistic effects with the other natural hormones covered in this book, particularly with thyroid hormone. Because of the synergistic effect of taking DHEA with the other natural hormones, I rarely use DHEA as a sole hormonal therapy.

Side Effects: DHEA

Side effects from using physiologic doses (mentioned previously) of DHEA are rare. The side effects I have witnessed have been acne and moodiness occurring in approximately 5% of my patients, usually young females. I have also noticed very mild hair growth occurring in 1% of my patients, a problem that is easily managed with reducing the dose.

Natural Hydrocortisone

Over 60 years ago, it was recognized that the use of thyroid hormone in the hypoadrenal patient could precipitate adrenal failure.[10] This can be prevented by combining small amounts of adrenal hormones with thyroid hormone, when indicated.

Hydrocortisone is a hormone produced in the adrenal glands--the same glands that produce DHEA. Adequate production of hydrocortisone is the body's major line of defense against stressful situations including infections and injuries. Without this increased production of hydrocortisone, the body is unable to adapt to a stressful situation.

When there is inadequate production of hydrocortisone, there is an increased susceptibility to illness (such as the common cold and other infectious processes) as well as longer recovery times and more severe infections from illness. In fact, adequate levels of hydrocortisone are necessary for the immune system to function properly and for the body to heal itself from illness or infection.

For people who have deficient hydrocortisone production, physiologic replacement doses (i.e., small doses) can improve the immune system as well as reverse many chronic conditions without any serious side effects. These positive effects cannot be achieved with the high doses (i.e., pharmacologic doses) commonly employed in conventional medicine.

Cortisone/ Thyroid Interactions

Hydrocortisone production in the body is directly related to the status of the thyroid gland. That is, in a hypothyroid state, hydrocortisone metabolism and production is usually low.[11] In fact, It is well known that hydrocortisone secretion from the adrenal glands is decreased in patients with hypothyroidism.[12]

Cortisone production can be low due to the effect of hypothyroidism inhibiting the pituitary hormones that are used to stimulate the adrenal glands. This inhibitory effect can lead to a hypoadrenal state.

Therefore, in a hypothyroid individual, it is important to balance the adrenal glands before using thyroid hormone. As previously mentioned, if the adrenal glands fail to increase their production of hydrocortisone when thyroid hormone is given, adrenal failure can occur. My experience has clearly shown that if a patient is hypoadrenal, physiological (i.e., small) doses of hydrocortisone should be given before starting thyroid hormone.

In individuals who suffer from chronic illness, I have found it necessary to properly evaluate the adrenal glands by measuring their output of hydrocortisone. It is impossible to effectively treat many thyroid and other autoimmune disorders without ensuring adequate functioning of the adrenal glands. Measuring hydrocortisone levels can determine whether the adrenal glands are functioning properly. Treatment with small doses of natural hydrocortisone (Cortef®), when indicated, has proven to be invaluable in helping these patients overcome their illness.

Autoimmune thyroid conditions, such as Hashimoto's and Graves' disease, respond particularly well to physiologic doses of hydrocortisone in the hypoadrenal state. When hypoadrenalism is present, chronic fatigue syndrome and fibromyalgia also respond positively to physiologic (i.e., small) doses of hydrocortisone.

Case Studies: Hydrocortisone and Autoimmune Thyroid Disease

Tom, age 57, was diagnosed with Graves' disease three years ago. He said, "Sometimes I feel as if I am in someone else's body. I have nerve tingling and weakness in my arms and legs. When my Graves' disease acts up, I often feel as if somebody turned up my energy switch too high. I can rarely relax." Tom was treated with PTU® (an anti-thyroid medication), which alleviated some of his symptoms. However, Tom also exhibited many of the signs of hypothyroidism including feeling fatigued much of the time. "I have gone from one extreme to the other— from too much energy to too little energy. I just want to be stable," he claimed. Tom's blood tests would frequently swing from hyperthyroid to hypothyroid. It was very difficult to medicate Tom with thyroid hormone because of the instability of his condition. When I checked a 24-hour urine test, Tom's results pointed to a hypoadrenal state with a poor production of hydrocortisone and DHEA. Tom was treated with 30mg of hydrocortisone per day and 5mg of DHEA per day. "From the moment I took the hydrocortisone and the DHEA, my body began to level out. I no longer had the severe swings of the Graves' disease. I was able to control the symptoms so much better," he commented. Tom was also able to take a daily amount of thyroid hormone, which significantly improved his fatigue.

Julia, age 36, was diagnosed with Hashimoto's disease one year ago. "I haven't felt well since I was a teenager. I had horrible PMS and I have always been fatigued. Over the last year, my symptoms have been much worse," she said. Julia kept asking doctors to check her thyroid hormone levels, but they always came back normal. "I knew something was wrong. I felt like my brain was only working at 50%. All the doctors kept telling me was I was depressed, and that I needed an antidepressant. I knew I did not feel well, but I also knew that I was not depressed," she commented. Julia had many of the signs of hypothyroidism including fatigue, cold hands and feet, dry skin, poor nail growth and hair loss. Julia's basal body temperature averaged 96.6 degrees Fahrenheit (normal 97.8-98.2 degrees Fahrenheit). Julia's T3 level was low, but her TSH level was in the normal range. She also had signs of hypoadrenalism including low blood pressure (86/50) and low levels of adrenal hormones. When Julia was treated with a small amount of hydrocortisone and thyroid hormone, all of her symptoms improved within two weeks. "I *couldn't believe the difference. It was like night and day. Everything that was wrong with me started to get better. After taking the hormones for two months, I felt 90% better. I now feel normal,"* she happily commented.

As mentioned above, physiologic doses of hydrocortisone are often necessary to support a hypoadrenal function in patients suffering from Graves' disease and Hashimoto's disease (as well a other autoimmune disorders). My experience has shown that small doses of hydrocortisone help the body utilize thyroid hormone much more effectively and help alleviate the symptoms of low adrenal function.

Natural Hydrocortisone Dosages and Recommendations

The possible side effects associated with hydrocortisone and other steroids include the promotion of weight gain, osteoporosis, arteriosclerosis and blood sugar abnormalities. However, I have observed no major side effects with the use of hydrocortisone in physiologic replacement doses--doses less than

40mg per day. The main side effect I have observed with taking a physiologic dose is a small weight gain, usually less than five pounds. Generally, this weight gain will subside after one or two months of taking hydrocortisone.

Natural Testosterone

Testosterone, like DHEA and hydrocortisone, is also produced in the adrenal glands. Testosterone is the main hormone produced by the testicles in men, with smaller amounts produced by the adrenal glands. In women, testosterone is produced in the ovaries and the adrenal glands. Women produce testosterone in much smaller amounts than men. Testosterone is one of the major regulators of sugar, fat and protein metabolism in the body. Natural testosterone, when used prudently, is a very important part of hormone balancing in both men and women.

There are two forms of testosterone supplementation currently available: natural testosterone and synthetic testosterone. Natural testosterone is made from plant products and has the same chemical structure as testosterone that is produced in the human body. Synthetic testosterone products, such as methyl testosterone, testosterone enanthinate or testosterone cypionate do not have the same chemical structure as the testosterone that is produced in our bodies. I have found natural testosterone to be very safe and effective in treating many different conditions, including autoimmune disorders. I believe natural testosterone, rather than a synthetic version, should be used in all cases of testosterone therapy.

I have yet to see a patient ill from autoimmune thyroid disease or another autoimmune disease that does not have significantly depressed testosterone and DHEA levels. Furthermore, these patients often have lowered thyroid and ovarian function. Most people suffering from autoimmune disorders will respond favorably to physiologic replacement of natural hormones, such as natural testosterone.

The Relationship between Testosterone and Thyroid Disorders

There is a close relationship between testosterone levels and hypothyroidism. Researchers have pointed out that in hypothyroid men, testosterone levels are unusually low.[13] A recent study found that hypothyroid men with low testosterone levels had their testosterone levels returned to normal upon taking thyroid hormone replacement. The authors suggest that low testosterone levels may be a contributing factor to some of the symptoms and signs of hypothyroidism.[14] Abnormalities in testosterone production have also been noted in hyperthyroidism.[15]

In my experience, low testosterone levels go hand-in-hand with hypothyroidism and hyperthyroidism in men and women. The simultaneous use of thyroid hormone and natural testosterone provides a synergistic effect for the body and helps to improve many autoimmune disorders. In other words, the best results are achieved when both hormones are used in combination rather than using the hormones individually.

Discussion: Natural Testosterone

I have found sub-optimal testosterone levels in my patients who suffer from thyroid and other chronic disorders, including autoimmune disorders. Testosterone, like DHEA, is an anabolic (i.e., muscle building) hormone that aids the body in repairing injured tissues in many chronic illnesses.

Although there are not a lot of research studies looking at the use of testosterone in treating autoimmune thyroid disorders, there is a host of research testing the use of testosterone with other autoimmune disorders like Lupus or rheumatoid arthritis. One study found that the use of testosterone significantly improved the symptoms in patients with Lupus. The authors of this study concluded that low levels of androgens, which include testosterone and DHEA were thought to play a role in the development of autoimmune disease.[16] I have observed similar positive effects using physiologic doses of testosterone as part of an overall hormonal balancing regimen in those that suffer from all thyroid disorders.

The discussion of testosterone brings thoughts of huge body builders taking anabolic (i.e., muscle and tissue building) steroids to artificially bulk up. When taken in extremely large (i.e., supra-pharmacologic) doses, testosterone does promote the growth of huge muscles and can even result in aggressive and violent behavior. In addition, large doses of testosterone can lead to the development of hypertension, baldness, acne and other deleterious side effects.

However, with physiologic replacement doses--small doses that will not shut off the body's own production of the hormone--these negative side effects will not occur. In fact, I have found testosterone supplementation to be one of the most beneficial and safe hormone replacement treatments for men and women.

As with the other hormones mentioned in this book, I recommend using the natural form of the hormone: in this case, natural testosterone. My reasoning is the same as previously presented. In order to get the maximum benefit from hormonal replacement therapy, it is important to try and mimic the body's own production of its hormones. When used appropriately, I have found natural, bioidentical testosterone to be extremely safe and effective, without any appreciable adverse effects. This safety record is contrasted with the use of synthetic forms of testosterone (methyl testosterone, testosterone cypionate, or testosterone enanthinate), which are primarily used in the United States. Methyl testosterone (a synthetic version of testosterone) has been found to be carcinogenic.[17]

Natural Testosterone Dosages and Recommendations

When supplementing with testosterone, I recommend only natural, bioidentical testosterone (not the synthetic derivatives of testosterone) because it more closely mimics the body's own production of testosterone. Doses for women usually average 2-10mg/day. For men, doses usually range from 40-120mg/day. I prefer to use testosterone in cream form, as it is well absorbed through the skin. I recommend USP grade, micronized natural testosterone, which can easily be made by a compounding pharmacist. For more information on finding a compounding pharmacist, please see Appendix B.

Side Effects: Natural Testosterone

Doses of testosterone that are too high can lead to the development of hypertension, acne, hair loss, anger, and mood swings. I have not observed any major negative effects with using physiologic replacement doses of natural testosterone. There is some concern that testosterone could adversely affect prostate cancer. Consequently, I do not recommend testosterone therapy for a patient who has had a diagnosis of prostate cancer. Taking an herb, saw palmetto (300mg twice per day), may block any possible negative effect of testosterone on the prostate by stopping the conversion of testosterone to dihydrotestosterone. Dihydrotestosterone is thought to cause the excess growth of the prostate gland.

Natural Progesterone

Progesterone is one of two major hormones produced by the ovaries in females (the other is estrogen). Progesterone is primarily produced in the second half of the woman's menstrual cycle and is the hormone necessary for the survival of the fetus.

Men produce very tiny amounts of progesterone in the adrenal glands and the testicular glands. In men and women, a small amount of progesterone is produced in the adrenal glands, where it acts as a precursor for the adrenal hormones: estrogen, testosterone, and cortical steroids (hydrocortisone). There are two types of progesterone currently available: natural progesterone and synthetic progesterone (e.g., Provera®). Natural progesterone is made from plant products and has the same chemical structure as the progesterone produced in the human body. For a comparison of the difference in the chemical structure of natural progesterone and Provera®, see Figure 1 (page 171). I have found natural progesterone to be much more effective and safer for treating illness and promoting health than synthetic forms of progesterone, such as Provera®.

Progesterone/Thyroid Relationship

Adequate levels of thyroid hormone are necessary for the production of progesterone in the ovaries. Both hypothyroidism and hyperthyroidism can cause problems with the production of progesterone in the ovaries.[18] Progesterone has the ability to facilitate thyroid function in the body and can be beneficial in both the hypothyroid and the hyperthyroid patient. Natural, bioidentical progesterone and thyroid hormone have a synergistic effect when used together.

Case Study: Natural Progesterone

Jill, a 52-year-old business executive found her declining health had affected her ability to work. "I need to be focused at work and I just can't keep things straight any more," she said. Jill first noticed a decline in her memory two years ago. This coincided with the onset of menopausal symptoms, which included hot flashes. "At first, I did not know what was going on. I would be driving somewhere, and I could not remember where I was going. Then, I couldn't remember talking with my clients. Needless to say, this is not good for my professional career," she claimed. Jill also complained of severe fatigue. She said, "I found that I could not get out of bed in the morning. I used to work out every morning, and now I find myself drinking a couple of cups of coffee just to get going." Jill was found to be hypothyroid and deficient in progesterone. When Jill was treated with both

Armour® Thyroid and natural progesterone, her symptoms rapidly improved. "It was amazing. I became my old self again in a matter of months. My energy returned and my memory came back. Even people at work were asking me what I was doing since I looked so good."

It is very common for borderline thyroid problems to become exaggerated during periods of stress. For a woman, this can include the onset of menopause or even the start of a menstrual period. Furthermore, I have found very good results with my patients when using natural progesterone along with thyroid hormone. These hormones have a synergistic action when used in combination.

Natural Progesterone: Doses and Recommendations

Natural progesterone is available in a cream form, which is absorbed through the skin and in a pill form. I usually recommend using the cream because its absorption appears to be better than that of the pill. There are several natural progesterone creams available in health food stores. My research has shown, however, that many over-the-counter brands of natural progesterone are not consistent; the strengths can vary from jar to jar. I have found better results with U.S.P. grade micronized progesterone, typically derived from plants and formulated by a compounding pharmacist. I use strengths from 1.5-10%, applied directly to the skin. Progesterone levels improve with this method; and, most importantly, symptoms improve. I recommend using natural progesterone the last two weeks of a menstrual cycle, and for three weeks of the month in a postmenopausal woman. Best results can be seen if progesterone is combined with thyroid hormone (and other bioidentical, natural hormones) when indicated.

Side Effects: Progesterone

The side effects of natural progesterone that I have observed include breast tenderness, moodiness and weight gain. These side effects are very rare and are usually dose related. These are contrasted with the adverse effects from the synthetic version of progesterone (Provera®). The side effects of Provera® include breast cancer, blood clots, fluid retention, breast tenderness, nausea, insomnia, depression and others.

Final Thoughts: Natural Progesterone

I believe Provera® is a very toxic drug. A recent study in the Journal of the American Medical Association showed that the use of synthetic progesterone (Provera®, Depo-Provera® and others) increased the risk of breast cancer by 800% as compared to the use of estrogen alone.[19] Furthermore, my experience has shown poor results in individuals with thyroid disorders who use synthetic progesterone drugs. Synthetic progesterone drugs should not be used for any condition. Synthetic progesterone drugs (Provera® or those found in birth control pills) can worsen any thyroid problem. Natural progesterone should be used for all cases of progesterone therapy.

Natural Estrogens

Estrogen is primarily produced in the ovaries. Estrogen is produced in a cyclic fashion in a menstruating woman. There are different types of estrogen manufactured by the body, known as:

1. Estrone or E1
2. Estradiol or E2
3. Estriol or E3

Estrogens have been used for hormone replacement therapy for many years. They are effective for treating the symptoms of menopause including hot flashes. Estrogens can slow down the rate of bone loss during the postmenopausal years and they can improve memory loss in selected patients.

However, there are growing concerns about the use of estrogen treatment. Recent studies debunk many of the proposed benefits of estrogen use, including the benefit of using estrogens to help prevent coronary artery disease.

A larger concern with the use of estrogen is the possible interaction of estrogen therapy and cancers such as breast cancer. Though there is no clear-cut answer to this controversy, I believe it is wise to be very conservative in the use of any estrogen therapies. However, the research is clear that it is the xenoestrogens which are a toxic form of estrogen. Xenoestrogens are synthetic estrogen-like chemicals that are thought to be responsible for the rise in hormone sensitive cancers such as breast and prostate cancer. Generally, we are exposed to many of these xenoestrogens in the environment from PCB's, dioxins and other chemicals. They are found in many household items such as plastic. These agents can lead to an estrogen dominant condition which may be responsible for the high rate of breast and prostate cancer. Therefore, I believe it is best to limit exposure to these estrogen-like chemicals and to undergo detoxification techniques to release these agents in the body (see Chapter 9 for more information about detoxification).

Estrogen/Thyroid Interaction

My experience with women using estrogen has been that a large majority of these women exhibit many of the signs of hypothyroidism. Researchers have found that increased estrogen levels may lower circulating thyroid hormone levels and inhibit the T4 to T3 conversion. Birth control pills that contain synthetic estrogen have also been found to inhibit the conversion of T4 to T3.[20]

If it is true, as previously stated, that we are living in a world of estrogen dominance, this may partly explain why there is so much hypothyroidism present in the western countries. I believe it is prudent to avoid taking synthetic estrogens, when possible. Birth control pills, in particular, should always be avoided. Also, if estrogen is to be used it makes sense to use natural, bioidentical estrogens. They are much more effective and safer than the commonly used synthetic estrogens (i.e., Premarin®) used in conventional medicine.

Joanna, a 22-year-old college student, suffered from fatigue for three years. "I am always tired. I could sleep anytime.

I have a very difficult time staying awake in school. It takes all of my energy just to go to class," she said. Joanna was a runner in high school. "Now, I couldn't exercise if I wanted to. I am just too tired," she claimed. Joanna was placed on birth control pills to control irregular menstrual periods five years ago. When I examined Joanna, she exhibited many of the signs of hypothyroidism including having poor eyebrows, swelling under her eyes, poor nail growth, dry skin and slow reflexes. She also had a low basal body temperature—averaging 96.8 degrees Fahrenheit (normal 97.8-98.2 degrees Fahrenheit). Laboratory work showed normal T4 levels but low T3 levels, indicating a poor conversion of T4 to T3. When I told Joanna that I thought her problem might be hypothyroidism exacerbated by the use of birth control pills, she couldn't believe it. "How could birth control pills cause such problems? They have sure made my periods better," she said. I informed her that irregular menstrual periods can also be a sign of hypothyroidism. After taking Joanna off of birth control pills, her T3 levels improved 30%. When vitamin (Vitamin B6 and Vitamin D) and mineral (magnesium and zinc) deficiencies were corrected, her T3 improved into a normal range. Furthermore, her menses returned to a normal cycle and her energy level improved. "I couldn't believe taking birth control pills could make such a difference in my life. I feel just like I did in high school now," she claimed.

I have seen many patients who developed hypothyroid symptoms or exacerbated a hypothyroid condition by taking birth control pills. Birth control pills are often prescribed for irregular periods, heavy bleeding and PMS (which are all signs of possible hypothyroidism). In addition, synthetic estrogens commonly used in hormone replacement therapy can cause hypothyroid symptoms. Because of the negative interaction of birth control pills and estrogens with the thyroid gland, I believe that these agents should be taken with the greatest caution and natural methods should be explored when available.

Human Growth Hormone

Human growth hormone is secreted by the pituitary gland, which is located in the center of the brain. It is named human growth hormone because its production peaks during the intense growth spurt of adolescence. Children lacking the proper production of human growth hormone will have an extremely short stature. Adults lacking human growth hormone have many signs of accelerated aging (increased skin wrinkling, decreased energy levels, poor sexual function, increased body fat, and signs of osteoporosis). Furthermore, accelerated cardiovascular diseases are common in adults with human growth hormone insufficiency. Thyroid hormone closely regulates the release and synthesis of growth hormone. I have found that people who suffer from thyroid disorders, including autoimmune thyroid disorders, often have severely depressed levels of growth hormone.

After the pituitary secretes human growth hormone, it causes the liver to secrete another hormone called insulin-like growth factor 1 or IGF-1 as illustrated in Figure 3.

Figure 3: The Release of Human Growth Hormone from the Pituitary

Pituitary Gland $\longrightarrow$ **Growth Hormone** $\longrightarrow$ **Liver** $\longrightarrow$ **IGF-1**

It is IGF-1 that is responsible for the effects of human growth hormone on the body. IGF-1 is easily measured in the blood and is the most common measurement used to assess growth hormone status. All levels of growth hormone mentioned in this book are measured as IGF-1 levels.

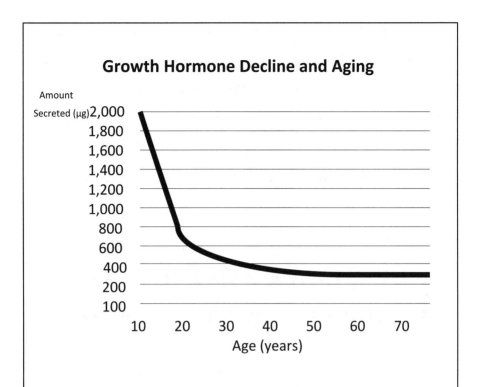

Figure 4: Human growth hormone decline as related to aging

In adults, human growth hormone production gradually declines as one ages, as illustrated in Figure 4. This gradual decline parallels the age-related decline of DHEA and testosterone. After the age of twenty, human growth hormone levels fall by 50% approximately every seven years. It is often the case that those who suffer from a chronic illness will have suppressed levels of growth hormone (as well as all of the hormones produced in the body). Perhaps by raising levels of human growth hormone (as well as DHEA, testosterone and the other hormones) to levels present at younger years, we can slow down or even reverse many of the signs and symptoms of aging. We may also be able to lessen the symptoms of chronic diseases such as chronic fatigue syndrome, fibromyalgia, and arthritis. Supplementation of human growth hormone does appear to clinically reverse many of the signs of aging in most people who take it.

Diagnosing a Deficiency of Human Growth Hormone

Human growth hormone levels can be adequately tested in the blood. I utilize IGF-1 as a good measure of growth hormone levels. I have found that effective serum levels for IGF-1 range from 150 to 300ng/ml in men and women.

Growth Hormone/Thyroid Interaction

Growth hormone and thyroid hormone levels are interrelated. Hypothyroidism has been associated with low growth hormone levels.[21] Thyroid hormone therapy has been shown to raise growth hormone levels. Conversely, growth hormone therapy can also improve thyroid function by improving

T4 to T3 conversion.[22] This again shows the synergistic effects of using combinations of hormones to treat illness.

I have found physiologic doses of human growth hormone to be safe and effective in promoting health, reversing the signs of aging and helping patients overcome illness.

The downside of the use of growth hormone is the expense: it can cost over $2,000 per year. However, there are other ways to raise growth hormone levels without using growth hormone. Exercise has been shown in numerous studies to enhance the body's natural release of human growth hormone. I have also found that the use of physiologic doses of other natural hormones (natural thyroid hormone, natural testosterone, DHEA, melatonin and others) can increase growth hormone levels. My experience has shown that using combinations of natural hormones enables one to use smaller amounts of growth hormone than would normally be used. Nutritional supplementation with amino acids has also been shown to raise growth hormone levels. In a study that I conducted, an interesting nutritional product, Gammanol Forte (manufactured by Biotics Research: 1-800-437-1298), was shown to raise growth hormone levels by over 45% in women.

Growth Hormone Dosages and Recommendations

Human growth hormone is given in injectable form. It is given in doses of 0.05-1.5 I.U. per day in a subcutaneous injection, which is similar to an insulin injection. It is best given in two divided shots per day, usually in the morning and at bedtime; this mimics the body's own rhythm of secreting growth hormone. Growth hormone, like all the other hormones mentioned in this book, should be used in physiologic (i.e. small) doses only. It can be measured in the blood as an IGF-1 test. I have found that effective serum levels for IGF-1 range from 200-300ng/ml.

Side Effects: Growth Hormone

One side effect of using human growth hormone is increasing the risk of acromegaly. Acromegaly is a condition where huge amounts of human growth hormone are secreted in the body resulting in a higher incidence of cardiac problems and premature death. Acromegaly is seen in athletes who take massive doses of human growth hormone and in other people who are born with a pituitary gland that erroneously secretes excess amounts of human growth hormone. I have not experienced any signs of acromegaly with the use of physiologic doses of human growth hormone.

Other adverse effects of human growth hormone include carpal tunnel syndrome, achiness in the joints and muscles, and edema. These side effects have been reported with high doses of human growth hormone and are almost nonexistent when using lower doses. Most of these side effects are easily reversible by lowering the dose. I have observed few adverse effects with the use of physiologic doses of human growth hormone.

Pregnenolone

Pregnenolone is a steroid hormone produced in the adrenal glands. Pregnenolone is often referred to as the 'mother hormone' since it is the precursor hormone to all of the adrenal hormones. It is formed from cholesterol and is necessary to produce other adrenal hormones including progesterone, DHEA, cortisol, testosterone, and the estrogens. Pregnenolone is also produced in the brain. In fact, pregnenolone levels in the brain are much higher than they are in the peripheral tissues.[23] Pregnenolone, like all the other hormones mentioned in this book, progressively declines as we age and is depleted in many chronic conditions, including thyroid disorders.

Pregnenolone is particularly helpful for fatigue states, arthritis, depression and memory problems. I have observed profound positive effects in my patients who have memory difficulties when using pregnenolone.

Pregnenolone/Thyroid Relationship

Researchers have found that pregnenolone levels are lower in individuals with hypothyroidism.[24] The authors of this study point out that low thyroid hormone levels directly cause the low pregnenolone levels found in hypothyroid patients.

The combination of small amounts of pregnenolone (10-20mg) with thyroid hormone has been very effective in helping hypothyroid patients recover their energy and improve their memory. Pregnenolone can easily be checked by blood tests and levels should be followed both before and after therapy.

Final Thoughts: Natural Hormones

Natural hormones are very effective and safe when used appropriately. A proper hormonal evaluation should be undertaken for everyone who suffers from a chronic illness.

Physiologic (small) doses of natural hormones should be employed to treat deficiencies. There is absolutely no reason to use synthetic versions of hormones when there are natural versions available. A natural product will work better in the body and have fewer adverse effects than a synthetic product every time. However, natural hormones should not be used without close monitoring by a qualified health care practitioner skilled in their use.

All of the hormonal systems of the body are interrelated and therefore the entire hormonal system should be evaluated in each individual. Consequently, treatment of one part of the hormonal system requires consideration of the other parts of the endocrine system. Natural hormonal therapies have a synergistic effect with thyroid therapies. When treating patients for thyroid problems, I have observed better results by assessing all of the hormonal glands and using natural hormones to achieve a balance in the endocrine system. Using an effective combination of natural hormones should always be the preferred protocol, rather than treating with individual hormones.

Furthermore, I believe in using natural hormones prepared by a compounding pharmacist rather than over-the-counter products because the compounded preparations are of a superior quality and contain consistent doses. To find a compounding pharmacist in your area see Appendix B.

For more information on natural hormones, I refer the reader to my book, ***The Miracle of Natural Hormones, 3rd Edition.***

[1] Jeffries, William. Safe Uses of Cortisol. Thomas. 1996.

[2] Barrett-Conner, E., et al. A prospective study of dehydroepiandrosterone sulfate, mortality, and cardiovascular disease. New. Eng. J. Med. 1986;315:1519-1524

[3] Gordon, GB, et al. Reduction of atherosclerosis by administration of dehydroepiandrosterone. A study of the hypercholeseteroloemic New Zealand white rabbit with aortic intimal injury. J . Clin. Invest. 1988;82:712

[4] Schwartz, AG, et al. Protective effect of dehydroepiandrosterone against aflatoxin B1- and 7, 12-dimethylbenz(a)anthracene-induced cytotoxicity and transformation in cultured cells. Cancer Res. 1075;35:2482-2487

[5] Van Vollenhovenm, Ronald. Arthritis and Rheumatism. September, 1994;37(9);1035

[6] Bassi, F, et al. Plasma dehydroepiandosteone sulphate in hypothyroid premenopausal women. Clin. Endocrinol.1980;13:111-113

[7] Tagawa, N., et al. Serum dehydroepiandrosterone, dehydroepiandrosterone sulfate, and pregnenolone sulfated concentrations in patients with hyperthyroidism and hypothyroidism. Clin. Chem. 2000. Apr;46(4):523-8

[8] Jeffries, William. Safe Uses of Cortisol. Thomas. 1996.

[9] Claebrese V.P. et al. "DHEA in multiple sclerosis: positive effects on the fatigue syndrome in a non-randomized study." In Kalimi M. Regelson W. The Biological Role of Dehydroepiandrosterone. De Gruyter. New York. 1990. p. 95-100

[10] Dluhy, Robert. Werner and Ingbar's The Thyroid. 2000. p. 815.

[11] Kenny, F.M., et al. Cortisol production rate. VII. Hypothyroidism and hyperthyroidism in infants and children. J. Clin. Enoocrinol. Metab. 1967;27:1616

[12] Dluhy, Robert. IBID. p. 815

[13] Wortsman, J., et al. Abnormal testicular function in men with primary hypothyroidism. American Journal of Medicine. 1987. 82. 207.

[14] Donnelly, Peter, et al. Testicular dysfunction in men with primary hypothyrodism; reversal of hypogonadotrophic hypogonadism with replacement thyroxine. Clinical Endocrinology. Vol. 52. 2. p. 197. Feb. 2000

[15] Velezquez, E.M., et al. Effects of thyroid status on pituitary gonadotropin and testicular reserve in men. Arch. Androl. 38(1):85-92, 1997

[16] Lahita, RG. "Increased oxidation of testosterone in systemic Lupus erythemaosis." Arthritis Rheum. 1983;26:1517-1521

[17] Nutrition and Healing Newsletter, Vol. II No. 12, 1995

[18] Maruo, T, et al. The role of thyroid hormone as a biological amplifier of the aactions of follicle-stimulating hormone in the functional differentiationof cultured porcine granulose cells. Endocrinology. 1987. Oct;121(4):1233-41

[19] Journal of the American Medical Association. January 26, 2000; 283:485-491

[20] Pansini, F., et al. Effect of the hormonal contraception on serum reverse triiodothyronine levels. Gynecol. Obstet. Invest., 23:133. 1987

[21] Chernausek, S.D., et al. Growth hormone secretion and plasma somatomedin-C in primary hypothyroidism. Clin. Endocrinol. 1983:19:337-344

[22] Grunfield, C., et al. The acute effects of human growth hormone administration on thyroid function in normal men. J. Clin. Endocrin. Metab. 1988:67:1111

[23] Sahelian, Ray. Pregnenolone, Nature's Feel Good Hormone. Avery. 1997

[24] Tagawa, Noriko. Serum dehydroepiandrosterone, dehydroepiandrosterone sulfate, and pregnenolone sulfate concentrations in patients with hyperthyroidism and hypothyroidism. Clinical Chemistry. 2000;46:523-528

Chapter 8

Diet

Diet

A balanced, healthy diet is necessary to provide the body with the proper raw materials that will promote healing and ensure optimum health. Sadly, most Americans eat an unbalanced diet that is not only deficient in basic raw materials (i.e., vitamins, minerals, enzymes, etc.), but also contains many toxic elements (i.e., *trans*-fatty acids, artificial sweeteners, etc.). This type of diet can contribute to poorly functioning hormonal and immune systems and can eventually lead to chronic illness. A poor diet also sets the stage for hormonal imbalances, particularly thyroid imbalances.

Food is intended as fuel for our bodies. It should provide adequate vitamins and minerals that the body can use to make energy and perform its vital functions. When we eat food that is devitalized (i.e., refined products), our body must use its own store of nutrients to break down the poor quality food. Devitalized food provides the body with an inadequate supply of nutrients that are vital for stimulating proper digestion. Constantly eating devitalized food will result in deficiencies of vitamins, minerals and other essential products and will inevitably lead to hormonal and immune system abnormalities.

This section was written to provide the reader with a quick reference for assessing and improving the nutritional aspects of their diet. Following these six steps will not only lead to improved health, but will also allow individuals to overcome thyroid illness. More information on how to implement a healthy eating plan into your regimen can be found in ***The Guide to Healthy Eating.***

6 Steps to Improving Your Diet

1. Eliminate Refined Sugar
2. Eliminate Trans Fatty Acids
3. Eat Organic Food
4. Drink More Water
5. Eliminate Artificial Sweeteners
6. Eat A Balanced Diet

1. Eliminate Refined Sugar

Today, the average American eats over 170 pounds of sugar per year.[1] In 1821, sugar consumption was estimated to be 10 pounds per person per year. In 1993, the average person was eating 145 pounds of sugar per year.[2] Refined sugar is devoid of nutrients which aid the body in the digestion of food. Consequently, when we eat foods that contain refined sugar, our bodies have to use their own store of nutrients to properly digest the food. Long-term ingestion of large amounts of refined sugar will result in our bodies becoming depleted of essential nutrients. The overuse of refined sugar will ultimately lead to multiple nutritional imbalances in the body, particularly B vitamin deficiencies.

The average American eats 20 teaspoons of refined sugars per day, which equals 16% of their daily caloric intake. With teenagers, the situation is worse; they consume 20% of their caloric intake as refined sugars.[3]

The increased use of non-water drinks has contributed to the increased sugar intake. Americans drink twice as much soda in 1997 as they did in 1973, as well as 43% more than in 1985.[4] Based on data from the National Health and Nutrition Examination Survey, soft drinks and other sweetened beverages now contribute the largest number of calories among all food types in the diets of the more than two thirds of Americans who drink them. Soft drinks now comprise nearly 14% of the total daily calories for those that drink them.[5] If those numbers are not bad enough, now soda vending machines are commonplace in schools. A 12-ounce can of non-diet soda contains approximately 10 teaspoons of refined sugar. Fruit juices are not much better than sodas. Water should be the beverage of choice (see section below).

Many illnesses have been associated with increased use of refined sugar (see Table 1).

Table 1: Illnesses Associated with Increased Sugar Consumption

1. ADHD
2. Arteriosclerosis
3. Arthritis
4. Cancer
5. Candida
6. Diabetes
7. Kidney Disease
8. Liver Disease
9. Thyroid Disorders
10. Tooth Decay

There are many sources of refined sugar in today's food supply. These include: corn syrup, fructose, dextrose, brown sugar, etc. It is wise to avoid these items.

There are many sweeteners that available that are not devoid of basic nutrients, including raw honey, black strap molasses, maple syrup and others. Also, raw fruits and vegetables can be used as 'natural' sweeteners in food. The consumption of fresh fruits and vegetables has dramatically declined in this country. The average American eats less than two servings of both fruits and vegetables per day. Fresh fruits and vegetables provide many vitamins and minerals that help the thyroid and other hormonal glands function normally.[6]

Recommendations

Eliminate refined sugar and processed food that contains refined sugar such as table sugar, brown sugar, corn syrup and dextrose. Use natural sweeteners such as maple syrup, raw honey, black strap molasses, date sugar and others.

2. Eliminate *Trans*-Fatty Acids

Fat is a much-maligned macronutrient. We have been brainwashed by dieticians and the diet industry into believing that eating fat is bad for our health and that dietary fat is responsible for obesity. What these 'experts' do not tell you is that there are 'good' and 'bad' fats. "Good" fats are an essential ingredient necessary for proper thyroid and immune system functioning. This section will show you how you can incorporate "good" fats into your diet to improve your health.

Fats are found in most natural foods. All fats can be classified according to their chemical structure. The following are the most common fats in our diets:

1. Monounsaturated fats (e.g., olive oil)
2. Saturated fats (e.g., animal fats, butter, coconut oil)
3. Polyunsaturated fats (e.g., flaxseed oil, fish oil, most vegetable oils)
4. *Trans*-fatty acids (e.g., margarine, candy, bakery products, french fries, peanut butter, etc)

Over 30 years ago, Dr. Barnes (recalled from Chapter 2) recognized the importance of adequate amounts of fat in the diet. Dr. Barnes knew that fat was a vitally important nutrient for a properly functioning thyroid gland. Dr. Barnes described how a diet low in fat would often produce symptoms of hypothyroidism.[7]

It has been my experience that inadequate intake of the "good" fats will result in thyroid abnormalities, including hypothyroidism. The Standard American Diet is devoid of "good" fats. Furthermore, the intake of excessive amounts of 'bad' fats such as *trans*-fatty acids will worsen (or can cause) any thyroid abnormality, particularly autoimmune thyroid problems (i.e., Graves' and Hashimoto's).

"Good" and "Bad" Fats

As previously mentioned, fats, like all substances, can have good and bad properties. "Good" fats provide the body with healing nutrients and help the cells of the body maintain their integrity. They are found in whole foods and are necessary for healing and the promotion of optimal health. Examples of "good" fats can include food that contains monounsaturated fats, saturated fats and polyunsaturated fats.

"Good" fats are necessary for many important functions in the body including:

1. Energy production
2. Forming the skin and coverings of the major organs of the body
3. Maintaining the cell integrity in every cell in the body
4. Providing the necessary raw ingredients for the body to produce hormones

On the other hand, "bad" fats poison the cells of the body and cause nutrient deficiencies, particularly deficiencies of the fat-soluble vitamins A, D, E and K. "Bad" fats are found in partially hydrogenated oils and are known as *trans*-fatty acids. *Trans*-fatty acids have been associated with a myriad of health problems including coronary artery disease.[8]

Trans-Fatty Acids

Trans-fatty acids are made by the hydrogenation of naturally occurring oils. Hydrogenation refers to the process whereby oils are reacted under high pressure and with high temperatures in the presence of a metal catalyst (usually nickel and aluminum). The remnants of both nickel and aluminum are present in the oils that have been partially hydrogenated. Both aluminum and nickel toxicity are very common in people with a chronic illness.

The hydrogenation process results in a chemical change in the oil, whereby hydrogen atoms are shifted to unnatural positions. These unnatural molecules are examples of "bad" fats. As a result of this conversion, the hydrogenated oil becomes a foreign substance to the body. Our bodies are unable to distinguish the hydrogenated product from the non-hydrogenated product. These foreign substances (*trans*-fatty acids) are actually incorporated into the cell membranes. This will disrupt the normal functioning of the cells of the body, blocking the utilization of essential fatty acids. This can lead to the development of many chronic illnesses, including immune system dysfunction and hormonal imbalances, particularly thyroid imbalances.

The end result of the hydrogenation process is the manufacturing of commercial products that contain a high amount of the "bad" fats or *trans*-fatty acids. There are estimates that, on average, adults in the U.S. consume 14.9% of their total fat as *trans*-fatty acids. Teenagers have been estimated to eat more than 26% of their total fat as *trans*-fatty acids.[9] Table 2 shows you common foods that contain *trans*-fatty acids with the percentages of *trans*-fatty acids in parentheses.[10]

Table 2: Average *Trans*-Fatty Acid Content of Various Foods

Bakery Products (from 30% up to 50%)
Candies (up to 38.6%)
French Fries (up to 37.4%)
Margarine (17%)
Vegetable Oil Shortenings (20%)
Vegetable Salad Oils (0-13.7%)

Trans-fatty acids are detrimental to our health. The deleterious effects of *trans*-fatty acids are shown in Table 3.[11] [12]

Table 3: Possible Adverse Effects of Consuming *Trans*-Fatty Acids

Adversely affects immune system cells
Alters cellular membranes
Causes liver problems
Correlates to low birth weight in human infants
Decreases HDL (good) cholesterol
Decreases levels of testosterone in male animals
Escalates adverse effects of essential fatty acid deficiency
Increases risk for coronary artery disease
Increases risk for obesity
Promotes insulin resistance
Raises LDL (bad) cholesterol

So How Do You Avoid *Trans*-Fatty Acids?

Avoiding *trans*-fatty acids can be difficult. Often food packaging is not adequately labeled with information concerning the amount of *trans*-fatty acids contained in the product. Although there are new regulations on food labeling, manufacturers still do not have to list trans-fatty acid content <0.5gm. Whole food may have fat in it, but *unprocessed* whole food has only a very limited amount of naturally occurring *trans*-fatty acids in it. Products that contain partially hydrogenated vegetable fats and oils contain a large amount of *trans*-fatty acids and should be avoided.

Recommendations

It is best to limit or, better yet, avoid *trans*-fatty acids. Avoiding products that contain partially hydrogenated vegetable oils will improve anyone's health.

3: Eat Organic Food

Part of the reason there has been such a rise in chronic illnesses in this country is due to food being contaminated with hormone-disrupting substances. A hormone-disrupting substance is any chemical that binds to the body's own hormone receptor and has hormonal effects in the body. These foreign substances generally stay in the body for prolonged periods of time, constantly stimulating the hormone receptors. Hormone-disrupting agents accumulate in fatty tissues of the body (e.g., breast tissue) and are very difficult for the body to expel. Natural hormones, on the other hand, are short lived and do not accumulate in the body. Hormone-disrupting agents are not only added to the food supply, they are also used in everyday life as common household chemicals, pesticides, plastics, etc. These agents are responsible, in part, for the rise in hormone-related cancers such as breast cancer and prostate cancer. In addition, many of these agents have been shown to disrupt thyroid function. Table 4 provides information on some examples of these chemicals. For more information on hormone-disrupting compounds, I refer the reader to the excellent book, **_Hormone Deception_**, by D. Lindsey Berkson.

Table 4: Hormone-Disrupting Compounds

Chemicals	Uses of Chemicals
Alkylphenols (BHT and BHA)	Act as a food preservative
Bisphenol A	Coat tin cans
Pesticides	Keep crops free of insects
Pthalates	Make plastic more flexible
Synthetic Estrogen-Like Hormones	Fatten animals

There are over 800 of these hormone-disrupting chemicals. These compounds wreak havoc with all of the hormone glands of the body, including the thyroid gland. Organic food should be free of all hormone-disrupting agents, including pesticides and antibiotics. Whenever possible, organic food should be chosen over conventionally grown food.

4. Drink Adequate Amounts of Water

The human body is composed of 70-80% water, with the composition of the brain being closer to 85% water. Because of this high concentration of water in the body, it is essential to have an adequate water intake to promote good health and optimal functioning of all of the cells. In fact, good health cannot be achieved without adequate water intake. Thyroid disorders, like all illnesses, cannot be adequately treated unless there is a sufficient amount of water in the diet.

It has been my experience that all thyroid conditions, from hypothyroidism to autoimmune thyroid problems can be improved simply by ensuring an adequate intake of water. Most people, especially those who suffer from a chronic illness, don't drink enough water. It is rare for me to see a patient with a chronic illness who does not have many of the signs of dehydration. The following are some of the signs of dehydration:

A. Fatigue
B. Dry tongue
C. Coated tongue
D. Vertical ridges on the nails
E. Dry skin
F. Poor skin elasticity

Many of the signs of aging, including the loss of elasticity of skin and muscles, are primarily due to the body's cells losing water. This water loss can be accelerated by many factors, including the following:

227

A. Inadequate water intake

B. Excess caffeine consumption

C. Excess soda consumption

D. Alcoholic beverages

E. Diuretic medication

Since water is such a nourishing agent for the body, it is important to drink water in its purest form, without additives and chemicals. Bottled water contains chemicals leached from the plastic known as phthalates, which are known to be hormone-disrupting chemicals. These agents interfere with the normal functioning of the thyroid gland and other hormonal systems of the body. Similarly, tap water contains chemicals very harmful to the thyroid, including fluoride and chlorine. Fluoride and chlorine have been shown to interfere with iodine uptake by the thyroid gland. The long-term ingestion of fluoride and chlorine, commonly found in tap water, is partially responsible for the increased incidence in hypothyroidism.

Recommendations

I recommend using a water filter that removes fluoride and chlorine as well as bacteria and parasites. There are many water filters that are worth investigating. An environmental laboratory that specializes in water testing can test your water.

To ensure an adequate intake of water everyday, I recommend that you take your weight in pounds, divide it by two and use this figure as the amount of water in ounces to ingest on a daily basis. See Figure 1 below. For more information on water as a therapeutic agent, I recommend reading the excellent book, ***Your Body's Many Cries for Water***, by F. Batmanghelidj.

Figure 1: Recommended Water Intake

1. Weight in pounds _____/2
2. Result is recommended water intake in ounces
3. Number of ounces_____/8=_____ glasses of water per day.

---

5. Eliminate Artificial Sweeteners

The United States leads the world in the consumption of artificial sweeteners by consuming over 50% of the world's production.[13] The National Center for Health Statistics estimates that two thirds of adults in the U.S. consume aspartame products and up to 40% of children up to the age of nine regularly drink soft drinks containing artificial sweeteners. 800 million pounds of aspartame have been consumed since its approval in 1981. This is equivalent to 5.8 pounds of aspartame per person per year.[14]

Aspartame is found in a wide variety of food products (see Table 5).

Table 5: Examples of Food That Contain Aspartame

Diet pudding
Diet soft drinks
Drug and Vitamin Preparations, especially children's preparations
(i.e., liquid Tylenol®, liquid ibuprofen, etc)
Hot chocolate
Laxatives
Many low-fat foods
Mouthwashes
Presweetened cereals
Presweetened tea
Protein powders
Sugar free chewing gum
Tabletop sweeteners (Equal*)
Toothpaste

Aspartame is the chemical name for the brand names NutraSweet®, Equal, Spoonful, and Equal-Measure®. Aspartame is a sweetener that is made up of three items: aspartic acid, phenylalanine and methanol.

Aspartic acid acts as a neurotransmitter in the brain. It helps the different cells of the brain communicate with one another. Too much aspartic acid in the brain kills brain neurons.[1516]

Aspartic acid also acts as an excitatory neurotransmitter. This refers to the ability of aspartic acid to excessively stimulate neural cells, resulting in an excess production of free radicals and, ultimately, the death of the neural cells. This can explain many of the neurologic problems seen with the ingestion of aspartame.

Finally, aspartic acid can cause hormonal problems. Hypothalamic lesions have been found in animals given aspartate.[17] Aspartate can increase the release of the pituitary hormones prolactin and gonadotropin hormones in primates.[18]

The second major component of aspartame is Phenylalanine, which is an essential amino acid. Phenylalanine is converted to tyrosine in the body, and tyrosine serves as a precursor for the manufacturing of brain chemicals that regulate food intake and influence mood.[19] Phenylalanine is particularly harmful to individuals who have a genetic defect in which they cannot breakdown phenylalanine; this can lead to brain damage. This condition is known as PKU and individuals with PKU must avoid foods that are high in phenylalanine, including aspartame.

Too much phenylalanine affects many of the brain neurotransmitters including L-Dopa and norepinephrine. Research has shown that increased blood phenylalanine slows brain electrical discharge.[20] An increased level of phenylalanine has also been found in Alzheimer's patients.[21]

The third major component of aspartame is methanol. Methanol is also a major component of antifreeze and is used as a solvent. Methanol is the substance that gives the sweet taste to aspartame.

Methanol is a very toxic substance that should not be ingested. One of the by-products of methanol degradation in the body is formaldehyde. According to the USDA, formaldehyde is a poisonous substance, even in small amounts.[22] Methanol poisoning (and perhaps aspartame intake as well) has been shown to cause a variety of problems including: peripheral neuropathy, pancreatitis, cardiomyopathy[23], cerebral infarction,[24] reduction of both blood flow to the brain and brain oxygen consumption as well as swelling of the brain.[25]

Aspartame has been documented to cause a variety of problems (see Table 6)[26]

Table 6: Documented Problems with Aspartame

Anxiety	Hyperthyroidism
Atypical or Unexplained Pain	Hypothyroidism
Brain fog	Increased Incidence of Infection
Breast Tenderness	Insomnia
Confusion	Liver Dysfunction
Depression	Memory Loss
Dizziness	Muscle Aches
Eye Problems	Muscle Weakness
Fatigue	Neurologic disorders
Fibromyalgia	Peripheral Neuropathy
Headaches	Restless Legs

Aspartame and all products containing aspartame should be avoided. Our bodies were not meant to ingest food that contains aspartame. As can be seen from Table 6 (above), the problems from ingesting aspartame are many.

My clinical experience has shown that patients with thyroid disorders (particularly autoimmune thyroid disorders) are particularly sensitive to aspartame. Dr. H.J. Roberts, an expert on aspartame toxicity, has also found a connection between aspartame and thyroid disorders.[27]

Aspartame is particularly toxic to individuals suffering from autoimmune thyroid problems, including Graves's disease, Hashimoto's disease and thyroiditis.

Gary, a 45-year-old pilot, suffered from numbness and tingling down his legs and occasional numbness and tingling of his arms. Gary had a long history of Hashimoto's disease and attributed many of his symptoms to Hashimoto's disease. Gary also suffered from a poor memory and could not lose weight. "I could not lose an ounce if I stopped eating. I exercise daily and I only get larger," he said. Gary was consuming four diet sodas per day (containing aspartame) and drank three cups of coffee per day with aspartame. I had told Gary to stop the aspartame numerous times. Finally, at one visit, Gary felt he had to do something. He said, "I couldn't go on. I had trouble concentrating at work, my legs and arms were going numb and I thought I was going to have to take a medical leave." After two weeks of going without aspartame, all of the numbness and tingling resolved. "It was a miracle. I couldn't believe how much better I felt. My energy picked up and my mind came back. I can't believe one substance could affect me like that," he said.

Gary's story is not unique. I encourage all of my patients to abstain from aspartame, but particularly those that suffer from thyroid illness. Aspartame is not the only artificial sweetener on the market. Others include: sucralose, acesulfane potassium, saccharine and others. I don't believe there has been enough research on the safety of any of these agents, and they need to be avoided.

Ellen, age 52, suffered with severe migraine headaches for five years. "I have been to numerous doctors and the only thing they can do for me is to medicate my headaches. The medications make me drowsy and give me side effects. I would rather have the headache than take the medications," she said. Ellen was also complaining of having a 'brain fog'. "I feel as if my brain does not work most of the time. I just can't think clearly anymore." Ellen had very low basal body temperatures, averaging 96.2 degrees Fahrenheit (normal 97.8-98.2 degrees Fahrenheit). Ellen's thyroid blood tests revealed a poor conversion of T4 into T3. Ellen was drinking three diet sodas per day and using aspartame in her coffee every day. When I counseled Ellen on eliminating aspartame from her diet, she couldn't see how this could help her condition. "I thought the artificial sweeteners were good for you since they don't have calories in them," she said. After three weeks of avoiding aspartame, she noticed an improvement. "My headaches began to go away. I couldn't believe it. It was like a vice had been lifted off of my head. I can't believe aspartame could do all that to me." Ellen also noticed an improvement in her brain fog. "I can now think so much more clearly. I feel back to my old self again." Interestingly, her thyroid tests showed improvement and her basal body temperatures also improved. Ellen was treated with a small amount of Armour thyroid® hormone, which further helped her recover her health. Today, Ellen still enjoys good health.

6. Eat a Balanced Diet

A balanced diet is essential in order to achieve optimum health and to overcome chronic illnesses such as thyroid disorders. An improper diet will not only result in a poorly functioning immune system, it will also inhibit the natural healing mechanisms of the body, promote obesity, and accelerate the aging process.

Proper choices of food will provide the body with the raw materials necessary to promote health, along with supporting a healthy immune system and a healthy hormonal system.

Hormonal imbalances, particularly thyroid imbalances, are more prone to occur when eating an inadequate diet. Eating the Standard American Diet, consisting of high amounts of refined carbohydrates, low-fat foods, and poor protein choices will, inevitably, lead to hormonal imbalances.

Food consists of three major macronutrients: carbohydrates, protein and fat. Carbohydrates are found in plant products and include starches and sugars. They are found in fruits, vegetables, grains, pasta, bread, cookies, alcohol, etc. Proteins are the building blocks of the body and they form the muscles and the organs. An adequate intake of protein is also necessary to produce hormones. Sources of protein include animal products (the most complete form of protein), vegetables such as beans and legumes, and seeds and nuts.

Fat contains more energy than either protein or carbohydrates, and it is essential for forming cell membranes and for hormone production. In addition, fat acts as a carrier for fat-soluble vitamins, including Vitamins A, D, E and K. Fat is found in animal and vegetable products. Vegetable fats are found in oils such as olive oil, flaxseed oil, corn oil, etc.

A sound diet must contain adequate amounts of good sources of carbohydrates, protein, and fat. This will provide the body with the necessary raw materials to promote health in the hormonal system, the immune system, and the entire body. The following section will help you to make the correct food choices to aid your body.

A. Carbohydrates

Carbohydrates are produced in all green plants in the form of starches and sugars. Glucose and fructose are examples of sugars. Carbohydrates are necessary for the body to transform fat into energy. However, the body has mechanisms to convert excess carbohydrates into fat. Sadly, the Standard American Diet contains too many carbohydrates and has made Americans the most obese people on the planet.

There are two categories of carbohydrates: refined and unrefined. Refined carbohydrates are formed from the processing of foods, a process which strips food of many of its vitamin and mineral components. The following are examples of ingredients and foods that contain refined carbohydrates:

1. White sugar and white flour
2. Pasta
3. Breakfast cereals
4. Corn Starch

5. Cookies, cakes, bagels, doughnuts and other baked goods

Eating these refined foods is very damaging to the body. Since these foods lack the vitamins, minerals, and enzymes that are necessary for proper digestion, the body must use its own source of vitamins, minerals and enzymes to properly digest these foods.

Overuse of refined carbohydrates can lead to a multitude of health problems including obesity, thyroid disorders and a host of nutritional deficiencies. In my experience, as well as what has been reported in the conventional medical literature, the increase in the use of refined carbohydrates has been directly associated with the rise in degenerative disorders as listed in Table 7.

Table 7: Degenerative Disorders Linked to the Use of Refined Carbohydrates

Arthritis	Diabetes
Autoimmune Disorders	Fibromyalgia
Cancer	Heart Disease
Chronic Fatigue	Thyroid Disorders

Refined carbohydrates also interfere with normal blood sugar regulation in the body. Refined carbohydrates are absorbed in the body very quickly and will result in a rapid rise in blood sugar levels. In response to the rapid rise in blood sugar levels, the pancreas will secrete a large amount of insulin. Excess insulin levels are an oxidant stress on the body and will accelerate any chronic disease process. In addition, excess insulin will cause imbalances in other hormonal glands, including the thyroid gland. Elevated insulin levels also deplete the body of a chemical called Cyclic AMP. Hormone synthesis in the body depends on adequate Cyclic AMP levels.

Unrefined carbohydrates are found in whole foods, such as fruits, vegetables and whole grains. These whole foods contain vitamins, minerals, enzymes and fiber that aid the body in their digestion. Therefore, the body does not become depleted from the ingestion of unrefined carbohydrates (in contrast to the ingestion of refined carbohydrates).

One must choose carbohydrates that do not excessively raise blood sugar levels. Dr. Barry Sears, the author of **_The Zone_** books, states, "All carbohydrates are not created equal."[28] Carbohydrates can be rated on a "glycemic index" scale. "Good" carbohydrates will have a low glycemic index rating: they do not excessively raise blood sugar levels. "Bad" carbohydrates will have a high glycemic index rating: they will cause blood sugar to elevate quickly, resulting in an exaggerated insulin response. A table listing of the glycemic index of various carbohydrates is found in Appendix A. There is no question that eating food with a low glycemic index is helpful to promoting a healthy hormonal and immune system.

B. Protein

Protein is the second most common substance in our bodies (second only to water). Adequate protein intake is necessary to promote general health and a balanced hormonal system. Proteins are the building blocks for all of the structural tissue of our bodies and are required to form the muscles, bones, nerves, arteries, veins and skin.

Hormones are synthesized from protein. Protein is found in animal products and in vegetables. Free-range eggs (eggs from un-caged chickens that are not fed any hormones or antibiotics) are a wonderful source of protein and should be eaten on a daily basis. Animal protein is the only source of complete protein available (i.e., containing all of the essential and non-essential amino acids). Vegetable protein, found in seeds, nuts, legumes and cereals, does not contain all of the essential amino acids.

Protein-deficient individuals cannot satisfy the body's daily needs for maintaining structure and repairing injuries. In addition, these individuals may also have hormonal deficiencies, particularly thyroid problems. I have diagnosed many patients with hypothyroidism that has been caused by an inadequate protein intake. Thyroid hormone is unable to convert from the inactive (i.e., T4) form to the active (i.e., T3) form without adequate amounts of protein intake (see Chapter 2 for more information on thyroid hormone).

Vegetarians must take special care to be certain that their diet is appropriately balanced with all of the essential and non-essential amino acids. Historically, humans have eaten animal products, augmented with vegetables, fruits and nuts. It is my belief that eating organic animal products (those that are free of antibiotics and hormones) is a safe and healthy way to provide the body with the necessary elements (protein and fat) to promote health and to have properly functioning hormonal and immune systems.

C. Fat

Eating adequate amounts of the right types of fat is essential to the production of all of the body's hormones, including those produced by the thyroid. Dr. Barnes (recalled from Chapter 2) recognized that it was necessary to have adequate amounts of fat (and protein) in the diet in order for the thyroid gland to function normally.

Fats, like all substances in the body, need to be properly balanced. This is particularly true with the polyunsaturated fatty acids. The typical American diet is deficient in good sources of both omega 6 and omega 3 fatty acids. I believe it is necessary to provide balance in these essential fatty acids in order for the body to produce adequate hormone levels. A fatty acid analysis can provide information to aid you in restoring this balance.

Not all fats are created equal. Many physicians and dieticians consider all fats to be a problem. However, eating the right kind of fat (one which is rich in nutrients) is important to provide the thyroid gland and other hormonal glands with the necessary ingredients to promote health. Fat is found in most natural foods. As described in the *trans*-fatty acid section, fat is an essential nutrient for your body.

Ingesting the wrong types of fat will ensure a poorly functioning thyroid gland and a poorly functioning immune system. This is also the case when ingesting low-fat food. Low-fat food leaves the body fat-deprived. A very low-fat diet or a diet high in the wrong types of fat will promote a poor immune system, a poor healing capacity and a malfunctioning hormonal system. It is best to avoid low-fat food products.

Katie, age 53, awoke one morning feeling very ill. "I had muscle aches all over my body and my feet were very painful. My husband had suddenly become ill the summer before and had gone through some difficult surgery and recovery. During this time I had not paid attention to myself. All of the stresses of the previous six months must have caught up with me," she said. Katie started seeing numerous doctors. "I kept being told all my tests were normal. I was told I had everything from arthritis to fibromyalgia to a nervous condition. I was given numerous prescription medications to take including Celebrex®, Vioxx®, antidepressants and anti-anxiety drugs. Each time I tried one of the prescriptions, I could not tolerate the side effects." When I examined Katie, she was clearly dehydrated. Her skin had a lack of elasticity to it, her tongue was dry and coated, and she had ridges in her fingernails. I also found her deficient in numerous vitamin levels, including Vitamin A and Vitamin D. Her thyroid tests revealed an inability to convert inactive thyroid hormone (T4) to active thyroid hormone (T3) and she had low basal body temperatures, indicating a hypothyroid condition. Katie's diet was also lacking in adequate amounts of protein. I made recommendations to improve her diet (eating whole foods, increasing fish) and emphasized the importance of eliminating artificial sweeteners, as well as correcting the nutritional deficits. "I added more protein to my diet and began eating wholesome organic foods. I also cut back my intake of carbohydrates and sweets. The effect of these changes was startling. My aches and pains are 90% better. My energy significantly improved, and more importantly, I now feel back to my old self." In making the changes in her diet and lifestyle, Katie's thyroid tests also improved. Her basal body temperatures also elevated to a more healthy 97.5 degrees Fahrenheit.

Final Thoughts

Eating a healthy diet can be difficult. Much of the refined food is inexpensive and readily available. It may take some work to change your diet to include whole foods and organic foods. I suggest that you try to follow the six steps listed at the beginning of this Chapter. Take it one step at a time and do not feel overwhelmed. Even small improvements in your diet can result in significant improvements in your health.

[1] U.S. Dept of Agriculture Report of the Dietary Guidelines Advisory Committee on Dietary Guidelines for Americans, 2000.

[2] From American Sugar Alliance website www.sugaralliance.org

[3] Nutrition Action Health Letter, Nov. 1998

[4] Nutrition Action Health Letter, Nov. 1998

[5] Spake, Amanda. U.S. News and World Report. 6.6.05. Accessed 11.17.07 from: http://health.usnews.com/usnews/health/articles/050606/6fitness.htm

[6] IBID Crazy Makers.

[7] Barnes, Broda. Hypothyroidism, The Unsuspected Illness. Harper and Row. 1976. P. 273

[8] Lichenstein, et al. New England Journal of Medicine, 6/99

[9] Enig, Mary. From web site, www.enig.com

[10] Erasmus, Udo. Fats that Heal, Fats that Kill. Alive Books. January, 1999 p. 103

[11] Enig, Mary . Know Your Fats. Bethesda Press. 2000

[12] Kohlmeir, L, et al. "Adipose tissue trans- fatty acids and breast cancer in the European Community Multicenter Study on Antioxidants, Myocardial Infarction and Breast Cancer," Cancer Epidemiol. Biomarkers Prev., 6(9) 705-710

[13] Bizzari, S, et al. High intensity sweeteners. Chemical Economics Handbook. 1996

[14] Roberts, H.J. Aspartame Disease An Ignored Epidemic. Sunshine Sentinel Press, Inc. 2001

[15] Olney, J. Brain damage in infant mice following oral intake of glutamate, aspartame or cysteine. Nature 1970;227;609

[16] Olney, J. Brain damage in mice from voluntary ingestion of glutamate and aspartame. Neurobehavioral toxicology 1980;2:125-129

[17] Olney, IBID.

[18] Roberts, H.J. IBID. p. 703

[19] Roberts, H.J. IBID. p. 687

[20] Elsas, L. et al. Changes in physiological concentrations of blood phenylalanine-produced changes in sensitive parameters of human brain function. Proceedings of the first international meeting dietary phenylalanine brain function,. May 8, 1987. pp. 263

[21] Shoji, M. et al. Production of the Alzheimer amyloid B protein by normal proteolytic processing. Science 1992;258:126-129

[22] Roberts, H.J. IBID. p. 673

[23] Monte, W.C. Aspartame: Methyl alcohol and the public health. Journal of Applied Nutrition 1984;36:42-54

[24] McLean, D. et al. Methanol poisoning: A clinical and pathological study. Annals of Neurology. 1980; 8: 161

[25] Roberts, H.J. IBID

[26] Roberts, J.G. IBID

[27] Roberts, J.G. IBID

[28] Sears, Barry. Enter The Zone. Harper Collins. 1995, p. 27

Chapter 9

Detoxification

Detoxification

One of the main reasons the thyroid gland can malfunction is from exposure to heavy metals including mercury, lead, cadmium, arsenic and nickel. These agents poison enzyme systems throughout the body and decrease the normal functioning of various organs and glands including the thyroid gland. Detoxifying the body and removing these harmful elements can vastly improve the overall picture of one's health.

We are exposed to a variety of chemicals and pollutants every day. These agents are in our food (e.g., pesticides), in our homes (e.g., household cleaners) and in our environment (e.g., petrochemicals). Our body must process all of these chemicals and remove these harmful substances from our system.

Our bodies remove toxic substances in a variety of ways including urination, defecation, breathing and sweating.

The liver is our largest organ and its primary responsibility is to remove toxic elements from the body. The liver utilizes a two-stage process that renders chemicals harmless, and then secretes them out of the body via urine or stool.

Problems develop when our detoxification pathways become overwhelmed as a result of overexposure to harmful chemicals. Exposure to harmful chemicals, as well as nutritional deficits and hormonal imbalances, can place a great strain on the liver and compromise the detoxification process in the body. Although this Chapter will primarily discuss heavy metals, there are literally thousands of chemicals that we are exposed to on a daily basis that can overwhelm the body's natural detoxification system and wreak havoc with the hormonal and immune systems.

When the detoxification process is overwhelmed, the liver is unable to remove these harmful substances from our body. These dangerous substances then begin to accumulate in different cells of the body. As more and more cells of the body accumulate these harmful substances, the cells begin to lose their ability to work and communicate properly. Consequently, malfunctions in the immune, hormonal and other systems of the body will begin to occur. A malfunctioning immune system sets the stage for chronic illnesses to develop such as infections, autoimmune disorders and cancer. In addition, a poorly functioning immune system will accelerate all of the signs of aging in an individual.

It has been my observation that it is impossible for someone to overcome illness and achieve their optimal health without optimizing their detoxification systems. I believe that every patient with a chronic illness should be evaluated and, when indicated, should be put on a detoxification program. This Chapter will explore various methods of detoxification.

People suffering with thyroid disorders often have poorly functioning detoxification systems. This Chapter will be divided into three sections:

1. Heavy metal toxicity
2. Nutritional support for aiding detoxification
3. Sauna therapy to enhance detoxification

Heavy Metal Toxicity

Heavy metals are a major cause of toxicity to the body's organs, hormonal system (including the thyroid gland) and the immune system. Examples of heavy metals include:

1. Mercury
2. Cadmium
3. Lead
4. Arsenic
5. Nickel

I have found heavy metal toxicity in a large percentage (>80%) of patients suffering from chronic illnesses, including thyroid disorders. In the case of autoimmune disorders, nearly 100% of my patients have laboratory signs of heavy metal toxicity. Is heavy metal toxicity the cause of the chronic illness in these individuals or just one of several factors inhibiting the normal function of their immune and hormonal systems? There is enormous individual variation in the accumulation and the sensitivity to toxic metals. However, the exposure to toxic metals will predispose the immune system to malfunction. My experience has shown that most chronic illness is a result of a number of factors, with one such factor being heavy metal toxicity.

Heavy metal toxicity can cause the thyroid gland to malfunction in a number of ways. In Chapter 3, thyroid hormone resistance was discussed. My experience has shown that heavy metal toxicity is related to thyroid hormone resistance. When the body is detoxified of heavy metals, the signs of thyroid hormone resistance generally improve. Patients are often able to lower thyroid hormone levels or stop taking medication when their body is properly detoxified.

Mercury

The U.S. Department of Health and Human Services lists mercury as the third most hazardous substance known to mankind.[1] The World Health Organization states that there is no minimum level of mercury that does not cause harm. The number one source of mercury poisoning is dental fillings. Dental amalgams (i.e., fillings) contain approximately 50% mercury as well as other metals, including nickel. The World Health Organization estimates that the largest source of mercury in humans comes from fillings implanted by dentists. The amount of mercury from fillings is over ten times more than for all other environmental sources combined.[2]

Mercury is also found in sources other than dental fillings. The following are some of the other sources of mercury:

1. Fish
2. Water-based paint
3. Polluted water
4. Fungicides
5. Some pesticides
6. Immunizations
7. Some cosmetics
8. Soft contact lens solutions

The American Academy of Pediatrics and the U.S. Public Health Service recently asked vaccine manufacturers to remove mercury from their vaccines. Mercury was put into the vaccines to act as a preservative. I believe that children should not be given immunizations with mercury in them.

A study recently released estimates that each year in the United States, 60,000 children are born with neurological problems resulting from exposure to mercury. Newborns can acquire mercury toxicity from their mother.[3]

Mercury is a known cell toxin that can cause imbalances in the immune system and can interfere with normal hormonal function. The thyroid gland and the pituitary/hypothalamic glands are very sensitive to mercury. Mercury is easily absorbed from the fillings in the mouth. It can be released as a vapor in the mouth, and chewing exacerbates its release. In fact, studies have shown that gum chewing can increase the release of mercury in the form of mercury vapor by 1,560%. Once released, mercury is easily absorbed in the body and concentrates in numerous tissues, including tissues of the following organs:

1. Brain
2. Kidney
3. Gastrointestinal tract
4. Liver
5. Fetal tissue (from the mother's fillings)[4]

Mercury is toxic to the body's own genetic material (DNA). Researchers have found a significant correlation between the amount of mercury in the body and the number of DNA aberrations.[5] In addition, mercury blocks enzyme functions throughout the body and decreases protein synthesis. Mercury exposure from dental fillings has also been linked to Alzheimer's disease and Amyotropic Lateral Sclerosis (ALS) by researchers at the University of Kentucky.[6]

Studies have shown higher mercury concentrations in the brain and kidneys of individuals who have mercury fillings versus those who do not have mercury fillings. Research has also shown a correlation with the number of fillings and the amount of mercury in the body. In addition, studies with animals have shown that mercury fillings can induce autoimmune diseases.

I cannot fathom why dentists still use mercury fillings when the danger and toxicity of mercury is a well-known fact. It is my opinion that mercury amalgams should be banned, as has been done in some European countries. If you suffer from a chronic disease such as hypothyroidism, Graves' disease, Hashimoto's disease, arthritis, chronic fatigue syndrome or fibromyalgia, you may want to have your mercury fillings replaced with non-mercury fillings.

Often, the removal of mercury fillings can be done gradually, as the fillings need to be replaced. However, the presence of a chronic illness will often necessitate a more urgent response. Whether you should have your mercury fillings removed should be discussed with a health care provider who is knowledgeable about mercury toxicity.

Mercury Exposure and Thyroid Abnormalities

Mercury has been shown to bind to the thyroid gland and disrupt its functioning.[7] [8]   Mercury binds very tightly to fatty tissues of the body (i.e., the brain) and to cells with sulfhydryl groups.   Many enzymes contain sulfhydryl groups that cause many crucial reactions to happen in the body.   One of those is the enzyme that converts the inactive thyroid hormone T4 into the active thyroid hormone T3—iodothyronine 5'deiodinase. Mercury has been shown to adversely affect this enzyme in fetal rat tissues.[9] Because mercury binds so tightly to our tissues and enzymes, the body has a very difficult time disposing of mercury.

Mercury has also been shown to poison the function of one of the body's main detoxifying enzymes—glutathione peroxidase.[10] This is one of the main enzymes that the brain and the liver utilize to detoxify the thousands of chemicals we are exposed to every day.

Selenium is a trace mineral that is very important for the thyroid gland to function normally (for more information about selenium, see Chapter 3).   Selenium is one of the most potent chelators (i.e., binder) of mercury.   Mercury exposure can lead to selenium deficiency. Selenium can be used up in the body as it binds to mercury in order to remove it.

The enzyme that converts the inactive thyroid hormone T4 into the active thyroid hormone T3 is an enzyme dependant on adequate selenium levels. Further adding to possible selenium deficiency is the fact that there is insufficient selenium in our food supply today.

It is vitally important that adequate selenium levels be maintained for any detoxification program to succeed. Appropriate screening tests including hair and serum testing should be done to check selenium levels and supplementation with selenium is important, when it is indicated.

Cadmium

Cadmium is an industrial pollutant. Cadmium toxicity can cause high blood pressure, anemia, and kidney and liver damage. It can also impair calcium absorption and influence the development of osteoporosis. Sources of cadmium include industrial waste, auto exhaust and cigarette smoke. It can also be found in some refined foods (especially white flour and rice), fertilizers, batteries, and sewage sludge. Cadmium exposure has been associated with thyroid abnormalities, including hypothyroidism in children.[11]

Lead

Lead is an environmental pollutant that is very toxic to humans. In young children, it acts as a neurotoxin and can adversely affect intelligence, concentration, and language development. Lead toxicity can lead to ADHD, headaches, fatigue, muscle pains, indigestion, tremors, constipation, and poor coordination. Lead is also a potent enzyme inhibitor in the body. Sources of lead include air pollution, bone meal supplements, water that has passed through lead pipes, batteries, lead paint, cigarette smoke, and hair dyes.

Arsenic

Arsenic is an environmental pollutant. Arsenic, at high levels, can cause many neurotoxic effects including headaches, drowsiness, confusion, weakness, and skin problems. It has been associated with anemia, kidney and liver problems, hypertension, heart failure, and skin cancers. Sources of arsenic include industrial pollution, insecticides, seafood, and auto exhaust. It can also be released into wells and ground water from underground mineral sources.

Nickel

Nickel is a heavy metal that is toxic at high levels but does have an essential role in the body at low levels. At low levels, nickel may help stabilize the building blocks of our bodies -- DNA and the RNA. In addition, small amounts of nickel have been used to successfully treat psoriasis.

Nickel can be ingested, inhaled or absorbed through the skin. Sources of nickel include tobacco smoke, dental fillings, dental appliances, industrial pollution, batteries, hydrogenated fats, fertilizers, and acidic food cooked in stainless steel cookware. Also, the manufacturing process for margarine and shortening requires the use of nickel. It is impossible to remove all traces of nickel from margarine and shortening.

Testing for Heavy Metal Toxicity

It is imperative that those who suffer with a chronic illness be appropriately evaluated and treated for heavy metal toxicity. I have found elevated heavy metal levels (especially mercury) in a large number of my patients who suffer from a chronic illness.

Heavy metal toxicity can set the stage for a chronic illness to appear, or it may be one of many items contributing to disease and poor health. In either case, the removal of heavy metals, through a proper detoxification program, can improve the function of the immune system.

An evaluation of heavy metals may begin with a hair evaluation. Hair testing has been shown to be a reliable indicator of the body's level of heavy metals. Hair testing is inexpensive and can provide additional information on the mineral status of the body. Hair testing, however, should not be the only method used to diagnose heavy metal toxicities.

Urine challenge testing has also proven to be a very reliable method to test for heavy metal toxicity. I have found urine challenge testing to be more sensitive and more specific than hair testing. Therefore, in those who suffer from a chronic illness, I believe a urine challenge test should be utilized to properly evaluate for heavy metal toxicity.

After taking a chelating (i.e., binding) agent, a urine challenge test is performed. The most common chelating substances used are DMPS and DMSA. These agents have a high affinity for binding to many heavy metals in the body. After the metals are bound by the DMPS or the DMSA, they will be excreted in the urine or the stool. (See the box below.)

Heavy Metal Challenge Test

1. Ensure adequate kidney function.
2. Check 24-hour urine for heavy metals.
3. Take a chelating agent (DMPS or DMSA).
4. Collect 24-hour urine output.
5. Check the urine for heavy metals.

DMPS is given by injection (3mg/kg of body weight). DMSA is given orally, usually in a single 500 mg dose. After taking either agent, urine is collected for six to twenty-four hours and sent to a lab for evaluation. The laboratory will report amounts of heavy metals released from the body.

Treating Heavy Metal Toxicity

Once a diagnosis of elevated heavy metals is made, an appropriate detoxification program should be implemented. Detoxification is necessary to allow the immune system to regain strength and to restore the proper functioning of the cells of the body.

A proper detoxification program should contain five steps:

1. Removal of the source of toxicity
2. Improvement of the diet in order to nourish the body
3. Use of the proper medication and nutritional supplements to aid the detoxification pathways
4. Consumption of adequate amounts of water
5. Sweating

Step 1: Remove the Source of Toxicity

As previously mentioned, the first rule of toxicology is to remove the source of the toxic agent(s). When a diagnosis of mercury toxicity is made, all fillings containing mercury should be removed before instituting a detoxification program.

However, caution must be observed when removing mercury fillings. If proper procedures for removing mercury fillings are not observed, there is a risk of actually increasing the release of mercury vapors in the body.

Proper removal of mercury fillings should be done with a rubber dam, and be performed by a dentist skilled in the proper removal of mercury fillings. Precautions should be taken to minimize the risk of mercury exposure to both the patient and the dentist.

After the mercury fillings have been removed, a challenge test should be performed to see how much mercury is still left in the body. DMSA and DMPS are examples of agents that have been shown to be reliable in testing for levels of mercury and other heavy metals. The challenge test was described on page 260.

Step 2: Improve the Diet

The second step in a detoxification program is eating healthy foods, which provide vitamins and minerals that aid the body in the detoxification process. I refer the reader to Chapter 8, which provides information on how to properly balance the diet with adequate amounts of protein, fat and carbohydrates.

In order to detoxify your body, it is necessary to reduce or, better yet, eliminate refined sugar from the diet. Refined sugar contains no nutrients and when eaten in excess will lead to obesity and liver dysfunction. Further, I recommend eliminating any intake of artificial sweeteners, including aspartame-containing products, as they are toxic to the liver. Natural sweeteners such as stevia or honey are acceptable.

Eating organic food is very helpful in any detoxification program. Pesticides on fruits and vegetables (also found in many juices) are extremely toxic to the liver and the fat cells of the body. Organic fruits and vegetables should not contain any pesticide residue.

Hormones contained in most conventional meat products have disastrous effects on the body. Not only are they an added substance the liver has to detoxify, but I also believe that many of these hormones add to the incidence of cancer, particularly breast and prostate cancer. These hormones also wreak havoc with our own hormonal systems. Therefore, I recommend that you eat meat from organically raised animals only.

In addition, organically raised animals have a more favorable fatty acid profile than do conventionally raised animals. In other words, it is healthier to ingest meat from an organically raised animal, rather than meat from a conventionally raised animal. For a healthier lifestyle, I recommend eating only hormone-free meat products.

Step 3: Take the Proper Medicine and Nutritional Supplements

It is essential to use nutritional agents that help clear the body's detoxification pathways. I have found that using DMSA (an oral mercury chelating agent) about one hour before removal of mercury fillings can be very helpful in keeping mercury levels low. Also, the proper use of nutritional supplements can assist in keeping detoxification pathways functioning optimally. This will help the body rid itself of toxins such as mercury. For a list of supplements recommended, see Figure 1 below.

Figure 1: Nutritional Supplements Recommended for Detoxification

Cilantro drops: 4/day
Garlic: 500mg/day
L-Glutamine: 3-6g/day
Multiple vitamin-mineral complex
Selenium: 400mcg/day
Vitamin C: 3000mg/day
Vitamin E: 800IU/day

Step 4: Drink Adequate Amounts of Water

It is impossible to properly detoxify the body without adequately hydrating the body. Water helps flush out toxins throughout the body, including the liver and the kidneys. Also, water can help carry nutrients into the cells.

It is best to drink most of the water between meals, rather

than with meals. To calculate how much water you should ingest, see Figure 2.

Water should be the beverage of choice. All sodas should be eliminated. Herbal tea is an acceptable beverage, but it is not a substitute for water. Finally, adding a pinch of unrefined salt (e.g., Celtic® Sea Salt) per day to the regimen seems to improve the body's utilization of water. More information on the use of unrefined salt can be found in **_Salt Your Way to Health_**.

Figure 2: Recommended Water Intake

1. Weight in pounds_____ /2.
2. Result is recommended water intake in ounces.
3. Number of ounces _____ /8 = _____ glasses of water per day.

Step 5: Sweating

Sweating is an important physiologic reaction in the body. Sweating allows the body to rid itself of toxic chemicals and clear the lymph system. Many individuals who suffer from chronic illnesses report that they do not sweat. I recommend using a sauna to help train the body to sweat. I have observed very good results with infrared saunas.

Research has shown the value of sauna therapy in stimulating the endocrine system. Sauna therapy has been shown to have a positive effect on the thyroid gland. Researchers found that sauna therapy can enhance thyroid stimulating hormone (TSH) secretion.[12] This could lead to an improved thyroid function.

Sauna therapy can have other direct hormonal effects. In Finland, researchers found that sauna therapy can increase the levels of human growth hormone (HGH) in the body.[13]

Perhaps the greatest effect of sauna therapy is the ability of the body to release toxic chemicals through sweating. Toxic chemicals such as PCB's can interfere with normal hormonal functioning and normal thyroid gland functioning. PCB's have been shown to lower thyroid hormone levels in rats.[14]

Sauna therapy has been shown to help the body release heavy metals. Mercury and nickel can be released in sweat.[15] [16] By reducing toxic metal levels, all of the endocrine functions will improve, including thyroid function.

I believe that sauna therapy is extremely beneficial in helping the body attain optimal health by releasing heavy metals and improving the lymph system. I think it is imperative for anyone struggling with a chronic disease to be able to sweat on a daily basis.

For those individuals who do not sweat, gradual acclimation to the infrared sauna is recommended. I recommend using the sauna for short periods of time at first (<10 minutes), and gradually increasing the length of time in the sauna. Usually after 5-10 sessions, the sweating response will be restored. In almost every case (from thyroid problems to cancer), an improvement in the individual's condition will be seen when their body can begin to sweat.

Infrared saunas are readily available and reasonably priced. I use an infrared sauna in my practice and I have an infrared sauna in my home. Information on purchasing an infrared sauna can be obtained by calling:

High Tech Health
2695 Linden Dr.
Boulder, CO. 80304
(800) 794-5355

Final Thoughts

I have included this section on detoxification because detoxifying the body is very important in overcoming chronic illness as well as helping one achieve their optimal health. Each individual has a threshold where a toxic element can begin to disrupt the normal functioning of the immune and hormonal systems. This sets the stage for disease to occur. In order to minimize the risks for illness, one must try to keep toxic elements at their lowest levels. We live in a modern world, which uses thousands of chemicals. It is vitally important to minimize your exposure to toxic chemicals and to institute proper detoxification programs to combat these elements. I have come to realize that it is very difficult to maintain good health without detoxifying. I recommend working with a health care provider who is knowledgeable about proper detoxification techniques.

---

[1] "ATSDR/EPA Priority List." Agency for Toxic Substances and Disease Registry. US Department of Health and Human Services, 1995

[2] Kennedy, David. Health Consciousness, 1992;13(3);92-93.

[3] Oakland Press, 7/12/2000, A-5

[4] Drasch, G., et al. "Mercury Burden of Human Fetal and Infant Tissues." European Journal of Pediatrics. 1994; 153:607.

[5] Verschaeve, L., et al. "Genetic Damage Induced by Occupationally low Mercury Exposure." Environmental Research. 12:306

[6] Hailey, Boyd. "A Study of the Toxic Effects of Oral Mercury and Bacterial Metabolites Produced in Periodontal Disease and Infected Teeth: Possible Relationship to Alzheimer's Disease." Presented at ACAM, 1999-2000.

[7] Nishida, M., et al. Direct evidence for the presence of methylmercury bound in the thyroid and other organs obtained from mice given methylmercury; differentiation of free and bound methylmercuries in biological materials determined by volatility of methylmercury. Chem. Pharm. Bull. 1990. May;38(5):1412-3

[8] Kawada, F., et al. Effects of organic and inorganic mercurials on thyroidal functions. J. Pharmacobiodyn. 1980. Mar;3(3):149-59

[9] Watanabe, C., et al. In utero methylmercury exposure differentially affects the activities of selenoenzymes in the fetal mouse brain. Environ. Res. 1999 Apr;80(3):208-214

[10] Watanabe, C. IBID.

[11] Osius, N., et al. Exposure to polychlorinated biphenyls and levels of thyroid hormones in children. Environ. Health Perspec. 1999. Oct;107

[12] Strbak, Vladimiu, et al. Effects of sauna and glucose intake on TSH and thyroid hormone levels in plasma of euthyroid subjects. Metabolism, Vol. 36, No. 5 (May), 1987, p. 426

[13] Leppaluoto, F., et al. Heat exposure elevates plasma immunoreactive growth hormone-releasing hormone levels in man. J. Clin. Endocrinol. Metab. 1987;65:1035

[14] Crofton, K.M., et al. PCB's, thyroid hormones, and ototoxicity in rats: cross-fostering experiments demonstrate the impact of postnatal lactation exposure. Toxoc. Sci. 2000. Sep;57(1):131-40

[15] Sherson, D.L., et al. Mercury levels of sweat. Its use in the diagnosis and treatment of poisoning. Ugeeskr Laeger. 1986;148:1682-3.

[16] Christensen, O.B., et al. Nickel concentration of blood, urine, and sweat after oral administration. Contact. Dermat. 1979;5:312-16

Chapter 10

Coagulation Disorders

Coagulation Disorders

This chapter will explore the concept of coagulation disorders and their relationship to thyroid disorders and other chronic diseases. In a healthy state, there is harmony in the body between two competing systems; the blood clotting system and the bleeding system. In a diseased state, there is an increased risk for disharmony between the two systems.

When the immune system of the body is not functioning correctly, as in an autoimmune disorder, this can lead to a hypercoagulable state. This means that the blood has an increased tendency to become thicker and perhaps form blood clots. In a hypercoagulable state, the blood literally 'thickens up' in the small blood vessels of the body. This results in a decreased blood flow to the muscles and other areas of the body that require a large amount of blood flow. This decreased flow of blood to vital areas causes difficulties with nutrient and oxygen delivery to tissues.

Muscle aches and pains are one of the cardinal signs in chronic fatigue syndrome, fibromyalgia and thyroid disorders. If people with these disorders exercise beyond what they normally do, frequently they have an exacerbation of their illness, including increased muscle aches and fatigue.

When a person exerts their body beyond what they are usually accustomed to, an increased blood flow is necessary to supply nutrients and oxygen to the tissues of the body. If there is a coagulation problem in the body, the muscles will not be supplied with an increase in oxygen and nutrients that they need. This can result in the muscle aches and pains as well as fatigue and weakness that are commonly seen in many chronic illnesses including thyroid disorders.

The end result of the blood clotting system is the formation of a blood clot. However, many individuals do not form the actual blood clot, but release fibrinogen and other substances that result in "thicker" blood and reduce the blood flow in the small vessels of the body.

My experience has clearly shown a relationship between a hypercoagulable state in the blood and many chronic disorders including thyroid disorders, particularly autoimmune thyroid disorders such as Hashimoto's disease and Graves' disease. In addition, other autoimmune disorders (e.g., Lupus, rheumatoid arthritis and scleroderma) as well as CFIDS and fibromyalgia often have coagulation problems present.

Many patients with these chronic disorders do not respond well to therapies that many other patients respond to such as thyroid hormone replacement, vitamins and minerals, etc. One theory of why these individuals are not responding appropriately to these treatments is that perhaps the blood flow to various tissues has been compromised due to the hypercoagulable state. This hypercoagulable state would prevent the flow of thyroid hormone, vitamins, minerals and other nutrients into the cells where it is needed.

One study found that 92% of individuals suffering from chronic fatigue syndrome or fibromyalgia had signs of a hypercoagulable state.[1] My experience in treating these disorders shows similar numbers. In addition, I have found over 50% of individuals with thyroid disorders, particularly Hashimoto's disease and Graves' disease have coagulation problems as one part of their illness.

How Do You Diagnose A Hypercoagulable State?

There are many blood tests that can evaluate the clotting system of the body. These blood tests include checking levels of:

1. Fibrinogen
2. Prothrombin 1+2
3. Fibrin Monomers
4. Thrombin/antithrombin

One laboratory in the United States has been instrumental in detecting coagulation disorders as part of the puzzle in individuals with chronic illness. They have been checking blood for coagulation disorders since 1983. I have found this lab a reliable testing facility for establishing a diagnosis of a coagulation disorder. The lab is Hemex Laboratories, and they can be contacted at:

Hemex Laboratories
2505 W. Beryl Ave.
Phoenix, AZ 85021-1461
1-800-999-CLOT

Why does the Coagulation System Become Activated?

There are hereditary factors that can predispose the individual to developing a coagulation disorder. Research has shown that approximately 25% of the population has an inherited tendency toward developing a coagulation disorder. One study recently reported that out of 400 patients with chronic fatigue syndrome/fibromyalgia studied, 83% had evidence of this inherited genetic tendency of developing a coagulation disorder.[2] My experience with treating patients with CFIDS and fibromyalgia also shows large numbers of individuals have a genetic tendency toward developing a coagulation disorder.

In addition to the inherited tendency, many other agents can trigger the coagulation system of the body to become over-active including:

1. Allergens
2. Bacteria (mycoplasma, chlamydia, borrellia and others)
3. Biological warfare agents
4. Chemicals
5. Fungi (candida)
6. Heavy Metals (mercury, lead, cadmium, arsenic and others)

7. Parasites

8. Trauma

9. Vaccinations

10. Viruses (EBV, CMV, HHV-6 and others)

When the body becomes infected with a pathogen (i.e., bacteria, virus, parasite), one way the body can protect itself from the pathogen overwhelming the body is to activate the coagulation system, thus depriving the pathogen of a blood supply and preventing its dispersal throughout the body. However, by preventing a blood supply to the pathogen, you also prevent the immune system from properly attacking the agent and destroying it. This can leave the pathogen in the body wreaking havoc with the immune system.

Other agents, (i.e., chemicals, vaccinations, allergens) can also set the coagulation cascade in motion, resulting in a decreased blood flow to various tissues and the signs and symptoms of chronic illness. In fact, anything that can cause inflammation can activate the coagulation system. I believe there can be a combination of factors, (viruses, bacteria, chemicals, trauma, etc.) that overload the immune system and eventually set off the coagulation system. This can result in the initiation of chronic health problems, including immune system disorders.

What about the Genetic Predisposition?

The patients who have a genetic predisposition-- 25% of the population-- cannot effectively shut of this coagulation system once it becomes activated. They continue to produce more and more coagulating substances (fibrin products) that result in decreased blood flow to all of the tissues of the body. This system is further accelerated in individuals with chronic illnesses including thyroid disorders.

Dr. David Berg, one of the foremost researchers on coagulation disorders claims, "As blood viscosity increases and blood flow is reduced throughout the body, the patient becomes hypo-this and hypo-that, such as hypothyroid..." [3]

Treatment for Coagulation Disorders

When a diagnosis of a coagulation disorder has been established, an individualized treatment program can be started. What must be kept in mind is that the coagulation disorder is one piece of the puzzle. It is not the underlying cause of illness in the individual. In other words, it may be the virus or bacteria that is setting off the coagulation system.

Therefore, the treatment of a coagulation disorder often involves using multiple modalities. Many of these modalities have been discussed in other Chapters of this book and they will be referenced there. These items can include:

1. Drinking water
2. Detoxifying the body
3. Treating pathogens
4. Exercising
5. Eating a healthy diet
6. Using anticoagulant herbs and vitamins
7. Taking Natural Hormones
8. Using anticoagulant medications

Drinking Water

Drinking water is integral to preventing the blood from becoming too thick and helping break up the fibrin-like products that develop. A dehydrated state will only exacerbate any coagulation problem in the body and prevent the body from healing itself. For more information on water, see Chapter 8.

Detoxifying the Body

Heavy metal exposure is known to set off the coagulation system in the body. I have found detoxifying the body an important step to reversing this condition. This can include the removal of mercury fillings, taking supplements and sauna therapies. Detoxification of heavy metals was explained in Chapter 9.

Treating the Pathogens

My experience has shown a large percentage of patients with chronic illnesses, including thyroid disorders, have evidence of infections playing a role in their illness. These pathogens must be appropriately diagnosed and treated. The infectious agents are one of many underlying causes of the illness. Treatment of infectious agents requires nutritional support, balancing the hormonal and immune system as well as using small doses of antibiotics, when indicated. This is explained in more detail in my book, ***Overcoming Arthritis.***

Exercising

Exercising can help increase the blood flow throughout the body and help the body clear itself of fibrin-like products. Exercise need not be strenuous; it can be as simple as walking. Water exercises are particularly helpful for coagulation problems as the hydrostatic effect of water can help improve blood flow throughout the body.

Eating a Healthy Diet

Eating a healthy diet is necessary to provide the body with the raw materials (vitamins and minerals) necessary to promote healing. A poor diet, on the other hand, will exacerbate any coagulation problems in the body. Chapter 8 details more information on a healthy diet. More information on eating a healthy diet can be found in ***The Guide to Healthy Eating.***

Using Anticoagulant Herbs and Vitamins

There are many herbs and vitamins that can help the body clear away fibrin products and help the coagulation system. Nictotinic acid has been shown to lower Lipoprotein (a) values, which can help in a hypercoagulable state. Enzyme therapies such as bromelain (from pineapples) and mixed digestive enzymes can aid the body in removing fibrin products. Herbs such as gingko biloba have also been effective. Vitamins, such as Vitamin B12, Folic Acid, Vitamin A and Vitamin E can help reverse coagulation disorders. Ensuring adequate intake of minerals such as magnesium, zinc and manganese also helps coagulation problems.

Nattokinase is an enzyme from fermented soy. Studies have shown nattokinase to have anticoagulation activity.[4] I have used nattokinase successfully for many patients suffering from a hypercoagulable state.

Natural Hormones

Testosterone has anticoagulation effects in the body. I have found improvements in coagulation disorders with the use of combinations of natural hormones including DHEA, pregnenolone and natural testosterone. Testosterone has been shown to have fibrinolytic activity and can improve hereditary factors of hypercoagulation-- lipoprotein (a). In addition, the improvement of thyroid problems significantly helps coagulation disorders.

Anticoagulant Medications

In addition to the natural items mentioned above, drug therapies can be essential in treating coagulation disorders. Heparin is an anticoagulant medication that has been widely used in medicine since the 1930's. Modern physicians use low-doses of Heparin to prevent blood clots, with almost no side effects.

Heparin is a naturally occurring substance in the body, found in the mast cells. Heparin can be found on the surface of almost every cell in the body and is found to be in high concentrations in the thymus, lymph nodes, lung and the skin.[5][6]

In many coagulation disorders, low-doses of Heparin can be very effective at helping to improve the coagulation system, sometimes with dramatic effects. Research has also shown Heparin can positively influence the immune system in a variety of autoimmune illnesses including Lupus, multiple sclerosis, renal disease, ulcerative colitis, migraines, allergic diseases and AIDS. In addition, I have observed good results with using low-dose Heparin, when indicated, in individuals suffering from autoimmune thyroid disorders, including Graves' disease and Hashimoto's disease.

Danielle, age 28, suffered with Hashimoto's disease. "Since the age of 11, when I started having periods, I can remember never feeling normal. I experienced tons of symptoms varying from small things such as dry skin to major things such as severe depression. I went through severe periods where I could not concentrate on anything," she said. Danielle suffered with daily headaches, monthly migraines, irregular menses, ovarian cysts, fluid retention, extreme fatigue, muscle and joint aches, brain-fog, as well as numbness and tingling in her arms and legs. Danielle went from doctor to doctor, until she was diagnosed with Hashimoto's disease. "It was a relief to get a diagnosis. I thought I would finally get better," she claimed. She tried various synthetic thyroid hormones without relief of her symptoms. When I saw Danielle, she was on Synthroid® and was still suffering from many hypothyroid symptoms. I diagnosed her with mercury toxicity and helped her detoxify her body. When I placed her on Armour® thyroid, many of her symptoms improved. She said, "There is no question that I felt better after detoxifying my body and taking the Armour® Thyroid, however, I still was not myself." When I checked Danielle for a coagulation disorder, her blood work revealed a hypercoagulation state. "When I was diagnosed with the blood-clotting problem, I was at a particularly stressful time of my life. I was desperate for some relief of my symptoms. Within a week of starting Heparin, I began to feel better. All of my symptoms improved at the same time. I have been on the Heparin for four months now, and this is the longest "up" period I have ever had in my life. I have more energy and feel better than I have ever felt. I have always wanted to be a physician, but I did not think I had enough energy to get through medical school. Now, I am sure that I can reach my goal of becoming a physician," she said. Danielle's laboratory tests all improved on the Heparin therapy.

How Is Heparin Given?

Heparin is given in injections, similar to insulin. Heparin has a short half-life in the body and must be injected twice per day. Through careful monitoring of laboratory tests, I have found virtually no adverse effects with using low-dose Heparin in my patients.

Jackie, age 66 suffered from fatigue, headaches and digestive problems her whole life. "Since I was a child, I never felt well. I was always fatigued. Sometimes the fatigue and the headache would be so severe that I wasn't functional for that day. I couldn't understand it. Other people around me seemed so healthy," Jackie claimed. Jackie went to various medical doctors who prescribed a variety of drugs to treat her symptoms, including anti-anxiety drugs. "The drugs were a big mistake. I did not need them and they did not work," she said. Jackie had been through many holistic treatments including using vitamins, minerals, herbs, relaxation techniques, etc., but nothing worked. When I first saw Jackie four years ago, I diagnosed her with a hormonal imbalance and placed her on a regimen of natural hormones including Armour® Thyroid, natural estrogens, natural progesterone, natural testosterone, DHEA and melatonin. "After finding the right combination of natural hormones, many of my symptoms improved. However, I still had my original symptom—fatigue. I was having more and more difficulty running my advertising business."

One year ago, Jackie had a retinal vein occlusion, which is a blood clot in the eye. She was told by her retina specialist to take an aspirin a day. When I tested Jackie for a clotting disorder, she had signs of a hereditary tendency to developing a clotting disorder and her blood tests indicated that her blood clotting system was in a hypercoagulable state. I recommended that Jackie stop her aspirin and begin Heparin therapy. "Initially I was in tears when I realized I would be injecting myself twice daily with something. After a long discussion with Dr. Brownstein, I felt better about the process and within two weeks, I started to notice a difference. It has now been seven months later and everything has changed. I have felt consistently good since starting the Heparin. I feel 'normal' now. I have no fatigue, I sleep better and my blood pressure, which was elevated, has returned to normal. I feel healthier now at 66 years old than I have at any time of my life. I find this extraordinary," Jackie claimed.

Jackie's case illustrates the success with using combinations of therapies to achieve the best success. Though many of her symptoms improved with balancing the hormonal system, Jackie had a significant improvement in her health when Heparin was given to reverse a coagulation disorder.

What about Other Anti-Coagulant Medications?

There are other anticoagulant medications commonly used in medicine today, including Coumadin and aspirin. The medication that is most effective for the clotting disorder depends where the coagulation problem is in the body. Generally, Heparin is much more effective than other anticoagulant medications. Your physician should be knowledgeable about the benefits of Heparin and can help guide you on the appropriate therapy.

Final Thoughts

Evaluating the coagulation system is a necessary step in anyone suffering from a chronic illness. A large percentage--25%-- of the general population has an inherited tendency to have a hypercoagulable state. Those with a chronic illness have an increased frequency of having a hypercoagulable state. Proper diagnosis and treatment of a hypercoagulable state can mean the difference between health and illness.

There are many natural therapies available to help treat a hypercoagulable state. This includes the use of enzymes such as nattokinase. To achieve the best results, I suggest working with a health care provider knowledgeable about how to properly diagnose and treat a hypercoagulable state.

[1] Berg, D., et al. Chronic fatigue syndrome and/or fibromyalgia as a variation of antiphospholipid antibody syndrome (APS): An explanatory model and approach to laboratory diagnosis. Blood Coagulation and Fibrinolysis. 1999:10.435-438

[2] Berg, David, et al. Retrospective study of 400+CFS/FM patients for immune system antibody production, activation of coagulation, and hereditary coag defects as predisposition for CFSIFM. Presented at International Society Thrombosis and Hemostatsis. July, 2001

[3] From ImmuneSupport.com. 10/05/01

[4] Clin Hemorheol Microcirc. 2006;35(1-2):139-42.

[5] Nader, HB, et al. Selective distribution of Heparin in mammals: Conspicuous presence of Heparin in lymphoid tissues. Biochem. Biophys. Acta. 1980;627:40-8

[6] Wright, Jonathan. Oral, low dose Heparin therapy for autoimmune and other conditions. Wright On-Line Newsletter. Vol. 1,1. Jan. 2001

Chapter 11

Iodine and the Thyroid Gland

Iodine and the Thyroid Gland

Carol, age 56, suffered with fatigue, headaches, constipation, and muscle aches and pains for years. "I can't even remember when I felt well," she said. Carol had seen numerous doctors and was finally diagnosed with Hashimoto's disease and hypothyroidism. She stated, "Before I was diagnosed, they kept telling me I was depressed and they prescribed antidepressant medication. I tried the medication, but it did not help." Although Carol was treated with thyroid hormone (Synthroid®), she still did not feel well. "Synthroid® helped somewhat, but I wasn't where I would like to be. The medication only helped with about 40% of my symptoms. The doctor kept telling me that my thyroid levels were normal and that my symptoms were not related to the thyroid. He wanted me to take a different antidepressant medication. When I asked him about checking my iodine levels, he told me I did not need iodine since there was enough iodine in salt. Furthermore, he told me that supplementing with iodine can worsen Hashimoto's disease," she claimed. When Carol saw me, I ordered a urinary iodine test. Her levels were very low--less than detectable limits as reported by the lab. I asked Carol to supplement with iodine at 50mg/day along with other nutritional items (Vitamins B2, B3, C, and unrefined salt) based on hair and blood testing. Within two weeks of beginning the supplements, Carol began to feel better. "It felt like a miracle to me. My mood improved and the aching markedly decreased. I haven't felt this good in years," she said. With the iodine supplement, Carol was able to decrease the dose of Synthroid® by half. Today, Carol takes 50mg of iodine per day, along with vitamin and mineral supplements and continues to do well.

Carol's case is not unique. Over 90% of patients test low for iodine. I have found it impossible to optimize thyroid function when there are suboptimal iodine levels.

This chapter will explore the relationship between iodine and the thyroid gland. Iodine deficiency is the number one cause of thyroid disorders. Although iodine deficiency was thought to be a problem of the past, it is occurring at epidemic levels in today's world. Approximately 1.5 billion people, about one-third of the earth's population, live in an iodine-deficient area as defined by the World Health Organization. This includes vast areas of the United States. In fact, in the U.S. iodine levels have fallen by 50% over the last 30 years.[1]

Iodine is perhaps the most important nutrient for the thyroid gland. The thyroid gland cannot make thyroid hormone without iodine. The two major thyroid hormones, levothyroxine (T4) and triiodothyronine (T3) each contain iodine as a major part of their chemical structure. The "3" and the "4" each refer to how many molecules of iodine are attached to the thyroid molecule. I have been researching and using iodine in my practice for over ten years. I have found it impossible to optimize thyroid function if there are inadequate iodine levels present.

One of the consequences of an iodine-deficient state is goiter (swelling of the thyroid). Nearly 200 years ago, it was shown that the cause of goiter was iodine deficiency and the treatment of goiter required the use of iodine. The U.S. added iodine to salt in the 1920's to decrease the prevalence of goiter. The amount of iodine presently added to salt (77µg per gram of salt)[2] does prevent goiter in the vast majority of people. However, my research has shown the amount of iodine in salt is inadequate for providing enough iodine for the rest of the body's needs. Furthermore, iodized salt is insufficient for maintaining proper thyroid function.

I have been testing iodine levels in my patients for over eight years now. I have found nearly 96% of my patients have laboratory tests indicating iodine deficiency. In speaking to physicians across the country, they are experiencing similar results. I believe iodine deficiency is the number one nutritional problem affecting a vast majority of Americans. Iodine deficiency is the main reason we are seeing such an epidemic of thyroid disorders including hypothyroidism, autoimmune thyroid disorders and thyroid cancer. These disorders cannot be properly treated if there is iodine deficiency present. This chapter will focus on iodine and the thyroid gland. For more information on iodine, I refer the reader to **_Iodine: Why You Need It, Why You Can't Live Without It, 3rd Edition._**

How is Iodine Transported into the Thyroid Gland?

Iodine is found throughout the body. In fact, every cell in the body requires and utilizes iodine. The thyroid gland contains the largest concentration of iodine—approximately 15-20mg when iodine levels are sufficient.[3][4]

The thyroid gland has developed an elaborate mechanism to concentrate iodine. The sodium/iodide symporter (NIS) is a transport molecule found in the thyroid gland that helps concentrate iodine from the blood stream. Other tissues of the body including the breasts, salivary glands, and the ovaries also use the sodium/iodide symporter to uptake iodine. In an iodine deficient state, the body will produce fewer sodium/iodine symporters. Conversely, in an iodine sufficient state, the body will produce more symporters.

How Does Iodine Become Incorporated into Thyroid Hormone?

Thyroid hormone is produced from an elaborate mechanism whereby iodine is bound to the amino acid tyrosine and incorporated into the thyroid molecule known as thyroglobulin. This process is known as organification. Don't be put off by the fancy term "organification". It simply means "bound to" something. In this case, iodine is bound to tyrosine and thyroglobulin in order to form thyroid hormones such as T4 and T3.

At the RDA for iodine (i.e., 150µg/day), there is enough iodine available to produce thyroid hormone and prevent goiter in the vast majority of people. However, the next section will show you why the RDA is inadequate to provide enough iodine for the rest of the body's needs and to prevent thyroid illness.

Does The RDA for Iodine Provide Optimal Amounts of Iodine for the Body?

The answer to the above question is unequivocally "**no**". The RDA for iodine does not provide the amount of iodine necessary to iodinate lipids and proteins which have many benefits including anticancer properties. The RDA for iodine is also inadequate to provide enough iodine for the rest of the body's needs.

There are many fat and protein molecules that require adequate amounts of iodine to become "iodinated". That means iodine becomes part of that molecule through a chemical reaction. This reaction is referred to as organification (i.e., bound to) and is illustrated in Figure 1.

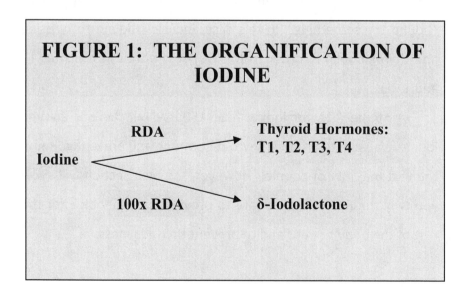

FIGURE 1: THE ORGANIFICATION OF IODINE

Iodine

RDA → Thyroid Hormones: T1, T2, T3, T4

100x RDA → δ-Iodolactone

As illustrated in Figure 1, the RDA for iodine provides enough to produce thyroid hormones which will prevent goiter. However, the RDA is inadequate to produce other organified iodine molecules such as δ-Iodolactone. Iodine is required in amounts of at least 100 times the RDA to produce these other crucial molecules.

Why the RDA for Iodine is Inadequate

From my previous discussion, the RDA for iodine provides enough iodine to produce thyroid hormone. Isn't that all the thyroid gland is needed for?

The thyroid gland does more than just produce thyroid hormone. It also produces other molecules such as δ-Iodolactone. δ-Iodolactone is a fat-like substance that is a key regulator of apoptosis and cellular proliferation of the thyroid gland.[5][6] Apoptosis refers to the programmed cell death that all of our normal cells have.

Cancer cells lack this apoptotic mechanism. They just keep dividing and dividing. One of the main thrusts of scientists who study cancer is how to enable cancer cells to become apoptotic. Iodine is one such molecule that has been shown to change cancer cells into apoptotic cells.

As previously mentioned, iodine levels have fallen 50% over the last 30 years in the U.S. One of the consequences of falling iodine levels that has occurred is the huge rise in thyroid cancer.[7] The incidence of thyroid cancer has increased 240% from 1973-2002.[8] I have no doubt this rise in thyroid cancer is directly related, in large part, to falling iodine levels.

How Much Iodine Do You Need to Ingest?

As can be seen from Figure 1, the RDA for iodine is inadequate to provide optimal amounts of iodine necessary to keep cells in an apoptotic (i.e., anticancer) state. Research has shown that 100x the RDA for iodine provides enough iodine necessary to produce the molecules, such as δ-Iodolactone, necessary to prevent thyroid cancer. This amount of iodine would be (150μg x 100=1.5mg) approximately 1.5mg. Is 100x the RDA for iodine the optimal amount of iodine?

Toxic Halogens: Bromide and Fluoride

The answer to the above question would be "yes" if we were not exposed to the toxic chemicals that further increase our need for iodine. There is a class of elements called halogens that contain bromide and fluoride. These items have become ubiquitous in our toxic world. We are exposed to ever-increasing amounts of these agents from our water supply which is fluoridated, to our food supply which contains brominated bakery products. Bromine is also used as a fire retardant and found in a wide range of consumer products including computers, furniture, automobiles, and carpeting. My research has shown elevated bromine levels in nearly all patients who have been tested. This includes both those that are healthy as well as those that are ill. However, those that are ill have significantly higher bromine levels as compared to those that are healthy.

Detoxifying from bromine and fluoride is essential to helping the thyroid, as well as the rest of the body, function optimally. Iodine is an essential ingredient to detoxifying the toxic halides. Chapter 9 will discuss the detoxifying methods helpful in allowing the body to excrete these toxic agents.

So, how much iodine do you need to take? I suggest getting your iodine levels checked and working with a health care practitioner who is knowledgeable about iodine. My experience has shown most people require iodine in daily doses ranging from 6-50mg/day. Those ill with chronic disorders may require more iodine.

Final Thoughts

This chapter reviewed the relationship between iodine and the thyroid gland. Iodine at the RDA ($150\mu g$/day) is inadequate to provide enough iodine to produce iodinated lipids such as δ-Iodolactone. At 100x the RDA, there is enough iodine to produce iodinated lipids that promote apoptosis. In the toxic world we live in, our iodine requirements have increased. For more information on iodine, I refer the reader to: ***Iodine: Why You Need It, Why You Can't Live Without It, 3rd Edition.***

[1] CDC.gov

[2] Venkatesh, M, et al. Salt iodization for the elimination of iodine deficiency. 1995

[3] Delange, F. Werner and Ingbar's The Thyroid. Lippincott Williams and Wilkins. 2000.

[4] Herzel, B. Modern Nutrition in Health and Disease. 1998

[5] Eur. J. of Endocrin. 132. 735-43. 1995

[6] Horm. Metab. Res. 26. 465-69. 1994

[7] Schneider, Arthur. Carcinoma of follicular epithelium. In Werner and Ingbar's The Thyroid. Lippincott Williams and Wilkins. 2000

[8] Davies, L. Increasing incidence of thyroid cancer in the U.S., 1973-2002. JAMA. Vol. 295. No. 18, May 2006

Chapter 12

Final Thoughts

Final Thoughts

This book was written to provide hope to those who suffer from thyroid disorders. Treating thyroid disorders is much more than simply adjusting medications based on laboratory tests.

This publication contains a lot of information. You may feel overwhelmed and not know where to start. This book will provide you with resources on how to start a holistic treatment program.

The information presented here has been gained from my experience in treating patients. I have seen positive results in using this holistic plan in my practice. By adopting this program, I believe you can share in the positive results as well.

The first step in beginning any treatment program is to educate yourself. This book was written to provide the reader with information about how a holistic program can be implemented to effectively treat thyroid disorders.

It is imperative for physicians and patients alike to realize the laboratory tests for thyroid disorders are not perfect. As explained in Chapter 2, thyroid laboratory tests may miss up to 40% of individuals who have thyroid disorders. The diagnosis of a thyroid illness is a clinical diagnosis, supported by findings in the history, physical exam, and basal body temperatures as well as the blood tests. This is a holistic way to diagnose a thyroid disorder.

Many times thyroid disorders can be corrected without the use of medication. Simply improving the function of the thyroid gland by taking the appropriate vitamins and minerals and detoxifying the body will help most thyroid disorders. Also, eating a healthy diet, as explained in Chapter 8 is essential to overcoming thyroid disorders.

If medications are necessary to treat thyroid disorders, my experience has shown that the commonly used levothyroxine sodium medications may not be the optimal choice. I believe that desiccated thyroid hormone is a more effective thyroid medication than levothyroxine sodium products. For individuals on levothyroxine sodium products (i.e., Synthroid®, Levothroid®, Unithroid®, etc.) who are not feeling well, a therapeutic trial with desiccated thyroid is indicated. For those with allergies to either corn or lactose, other options for thyroid hormone replacement are discussed in Chapter 4.

The role of iodine and the thyroid gland is discussed in Chapter 11. I cannot emphasize it enough: It is impossible for the thyroid gland to optimally function if there is iodine deficiency present.

There is hope for individuals with thyroid and other disorders. Don't accept disease. Educate yourself about the illness and search for answers. You must be your own advocate in the health care field.

This book can help you find your pathway to good health. I believe it is imperative to work with a health care provider who will consider your needs. If your doctor is not meeting your needs, I suggest trying to find another doctor. Appendix B will provide you with a resource of physicians who are trained in the natural approaches outlined in this book.

The information presented in this book will point out the safe and natural therapies that I have found effective to overcome thyroid disorders. Using the holistic approach outlined in this book will help you achieve your optimal health.

TO ALL OF OUR HEALTH!

Appendix A: Glycemic Index of Carbohydrates

The glycemic index is a measure of the speed of entry of carbohydrates into the bloodstream. Since carbohydrates cause blood sugar to rise, resulting in an elevated insulin level, it is recommended to limit the foods with the highest glycemic index and to eat foods with the lowest glycemic index (i.e. those with an index <50%).

High glycemic index, greater than 100% ('Bad' carbohydrates)
Grain-Based Foods
- Puffed rice
- Corn flakes
- Puffed wheat
- Millet
- Instant rice
- Instant potato
- Microwave Potato
- French bread

Simple Sugars
- Maltose
- Glucose

Snacks
- Tofu ice cream
- Puffed-rice cakes

Glycemic Index Standard = 100%
White Bread

Glycemic Index between 80 and 100%
Grain-based foods
- Grapenuts
- Whole wheat bread
- Rolled oats

- Oat bran
- Instant mashed potatoes

White rice
Brown rice
Muesli
Shredded wheat
Vegetables
Carrots
Parsnips
Corn
Fruits
Banana
Raisins
Apricots
Papaya
Mango
Snacks
Ice cream (low fat)
Corn chips
Rye crisps

Glycemic index between 50 and 80%
Grain-based foods
Spaghetti (white)
Spaghetti (whole wheat)
Pasta, other
Pumpernickel bread
All-bran cereal
Fruits
Orange
Orange juice
Vegetables
Peas
Pinto beans
Garbanzo beans
Kidney beans (canned)
Baked beans
Navy beans
Simple sugars
Lactose
Sucrose

Glycemic index between 30 and 50%
Grain based foods
Barley
Oatmeal (slow cooking)
Whole grain bread
Fruits
Apple
Apple juice
Applesauce
Pears
Grapes
Peaches
Vegetables
Kidney Beans (fresh)
Lentils
Black-eyed peas
Chick-peas
Lima beans
Tomato soup
Peas
Dairy Products
Ice cream (high fat)
Milk
Yogurt

Glycemic index less than 30% ('Good' carbohydrates)
Fruits
Cherries
Plums
Grapefruit
Simple sugars
Fructose
Vegetables
Soy beans
Nuts
Peanuts and other nuts

Appendix B: How to Find a Physician

For information on how to find a physician knowledgeable about using a holistic plan to treat thyroid and other endocrine disorders, you can contact the following two organizations:

1. Broda O. Barnes, M.D. Research Foundation
   P.O. Box 98
   Trumbull, CT 06611
   (203) 261-2101
   www.brodabarnes.org

2. American College for the Advancement in Medicine
   23121 Verdugo Dr.
   Ste. 204
   Laguna Hills, CA 92653
   (800) 532-3688
   www.acam.org

How to Find a Compounding Pharmacist

To find a compounding pharmacist, contact the International Academy of Compounding Pharmacists at:

The International Academy of Compounding
Pharmacists (IACP)
P.O. Box 1365
Sugar Land, TX 77487
iacpinfo@iacprx.org
(800)-927-4227
Fax: 281-495-0602

Index

Books by David Brownstein, M.D.
(For more information: www.drbrownstein.com)

IODINE: WHY YOU NEED IT, WHY YOU CAN'T LIVE WITHOUT IT, 3rd EDITION 2008

Iodine is the most misunderstood nutrient. Dr. Brownstein shows you the benefit of supplementing with iodine. Iodine deficiency is rampant. Iodine deficiency is a world-wide problem and is at near epidemic levels in the United States. Most people wrongly assume that you get enough iodine from iodized salt. Dr. Brownstein convincingly shows you why it is vitally important to get your iodine levels measured. He shows you how iodine deficiency is related to:

- Breast cancer
- Hypothyroidism and Graves' disease
- Autoimmune illnesses
- Chronic Fatigue and Fibromyalgia
- Cancer of the prostate, ovaries and much more!

DRUGS THAT DON'T WORK and NATURAL THERAPIES THAT DO 2007

This book will show you why the most commonly prescribed drugs may not be your best choice. Dr. Brownstein shows why drugs have so many adverse effects. The following conditions are covered in this book: high cholesterol levels, depression, GERD and reflux esophagitis, osteoporosis, inflammation and hormone imbalances. He also gives examples of natural substances that can help the body heal.
See why the following drugs need to be avoided:

- Cholesterol-lowering drugs (statins such as Lipitor, Zocor, Mevacor, and Crestor)
- Antidepressant drugs (SSRI's such as Prozac, Zoloft, Celexa, Paxil)
- Antacid drugs (H-2 blockers and PPI's such as Nexium, Prilosec, and Zantac)
- Osteoporosis drugs (Bisphosphonates such as Fosomax and Actonel, Zometa, and Boniva)
- Anti-inflammatory drugs (Celebrex, Vioxx, Motrin, Naprosyn, etc)
- Synthetic Hormones (Provera and Estrogen)

SALT YOUR WAY TO HEALTH 2006

Dr. Brownstein dispels many of the myths of salt. Salt is bad for you. Salt causes hypertension. These are just a few of the myths Dr. Brownstein tackles in this book. He shows you how the right kind of salt--unrefined salt--can have a remarkable health benefit to the body. Refined salt is a toxic, devitalized substance for the body. Unrefined salt is a necessary ingredient for achieving your optimal health. See how adding unrefined salt to your diet can help you:

- Maintain a normal blood pressure
- Balance your hormones
- Optimize your immune system
- Lower your risk for heart disease
- Overcome chronic illness

THE MIRACLE OF NATURAL HORMONES, 3RD EDITION 2003

Optimal health cannot be achieved with an imbalanced hormonal system. Dr. Brownstein's research on bioidentical hormones provides the reader with a plethora of information on the benefits of balancing the hormonal system with bioidentical, natural hormones. This book is in its third edition. This book gives actual case studies of the benefits of natural hormones.

See how balancing the hormonal system can help:

- Arthritis and autoimmune disorders
- Chronic fatigue syndrome and fibromyalgia
- Heart disease
- Hypothyroidism
- Menopausal symptoms
- And much more!

OVERCOMING ARTHRITIS 2001

Dr. Brownstein shows you how a holistic approach can help you overcome arthritis, fibromyalgia, chromic fatigue syndrome, and other conditions. This approach encompasses the use of:

- Allergy elimination
- Detoxification
- Diet
- Natural, bioidentical hormones
- Vitamins and minerals
- Water

THE GUIDE TO HEALTHY EATING 2006

Which food do you buy? Where to shop? How do you prepare food? This book will answer all of these questions and much more. Dr. Brownstein co-wrote this book with his nutritionist, Sheryl Shenefelt, C.N. Eating the healthiest way is the most important thing you can do. This book contains recipes and information on how best to feed your family. See how eating a healthier diet can help you:

- Avoid chronic illness
- Enhance your immune system
- Improve your family's nutrition

THE GUIDE TO A GLUTEN-FREE DIET 2008

What would you say if 16% of the population (1/6) had a serious, life-threatening illness that was only being diagnosed correctly only 3% of the time? Gluten-sensitivity is the most frequently missed diagnosis in the U.S. This book will show how you can incorporate a healthier lifestyle by becoming gluten-free.

- Why you should become gluten-free
- What illnesses are associated with gluten sensitivity
- How to shop and cook gluten-free
- Where to find gluten-free resources